MYOTONIC DYSTROPHY

the**facts**

A book for Patients and Families

Peter S. Harper

Oxford   New York   Tokyo

OXFORD UNIVERSITY PRESS

2002

OXFORD
UNIVERSITY PRESS

Great Clarendon Street, Oxford OX2 6DP

Oxford University Press is a department of the University of Oxford.
It furthers the University's objective of excellence in research,
scholarship, and education by publishing worldwide in

Oxford   New York
Auckland   Bangkok   Buenos   Aires   Cape Town   Chennai
Dar es   Salaam   Delhi   Hong Kong   Istanbul   Karachi   Kolkata
Kuala Lumpur   Madrid   Melbourne   Mexico City   Mumbai   Nairobi
São Paulo   Shanghai   Taipei   Tokyo   Toronto

and an associated company in Berlin

Oxford is a registered trade mark of Oxford University Press
in the UK and in certain other countries

Published in the United States
by Oxford University Press Inc., New York

© Peter Harper, 2002

The moral rights of the author have been asserted

Database right Oxford University Press (maker)

First published 2002

A catalogue record for this title is available from the British Library

Library of Congress Cataloging in Publication Data
(Data available)

ISBN   0 19 852586 9 (Pbk)

10   9   8   7   6   5   4   3   2   1

Typeset by Integra Software Services Pvt., Ltd, Pondicherry, India
Printed in Great Britain
on acid-free paper by
Biddles Ltd, Guildford & King's Lynn

Dedication

To the Myotonic Dystrophy Support Group, whose
work has helped so many patients and their families in
the UK and beyond.

*All royalties from sales of this book will be donated to the
Myotonic Dystrophy Support Group and the Muscular Dystrophy
Campaign.*

Preface

The idea of writing this book came to me shortly after finishing the 3rd edition of my larger book, *Myotonic dystrophy*. This was written for professionals, mainly doctors and scientists, but when earlier editions appeared, a number of patients and family members told me that they had found parts of it helpful for themselves. Now that this book was completed (after a long delay), I was conscious that there was a need for something written more specifically for families with myotonic dystrophy themselves, so I thought that I should try to provide this.

It could be argued that the Internet and information provided from other sources would make a book of this type unnecessary, but I rather doubt this. Perhaps I am old fashioned, but there are real advantages in having most of the information needed gathered together in solid form as a book, especially if it is short and easy to read.

The timing seemed good, since I had most of the details in my head already from working on the larger book, and the proofs of this were at hand. I also had the opportunity of a break on a remote island off the coast of Wales, free from telephone, electricity, and all the other encumbrances and interruptions of modern life.

So, with a background only of sea, seals, and birds to accompany the peace and quiet, I have written this short book, and I hope that patients with myotonic dystrophy and their family members, may find it helpful.

Peter Harper

Ynys Ennlli, Bardsey Island

Summer 2001

Acknowledgements

I should like to thank all my Cardiff colleagues, especially Dr Mark Rogers, for their help and support. I am particularly grateful to Margaret Bowler, Shannon Lord, and Maggie Wahl for valuable comments on the manuscript and for suggesting additional material, and to Michele Matthews for typing and organizing the text.

Thanks are also due to the Muscular Dystrophy Campaign (UK), to MDA, AFM, and to the Myotonic Dystrophy Support Group for financial support of the Cardiff Muscular Dystrophy Centre over many years.

MYOTONIC DYSTROPHY

the**facts**

CONTENTS

1
What is myotonic dystrophy?

Some information for those who know nothing or almost nothing about it

Most people who start to read this book will know little or nothing about myotonic dystrophy. They may have just been diagnosed as having it, or they may have learned that someone in their family is affected, but they will have only a hazy idea as to what the implications are for themselves. If this applies to you, this chapter is a good starting point. If you already have a fair amount of information, you can move on to the later chapters.

Why the name?

Fortunately, unlike many other medical disorders, *myotonic dystrophy* is a name that is reasonably easy to remember and to explain. The term *myotonia* is used for muscle stiffness of a special kind, while *dystrophy* is the name for any inherited muscle disorder in which muscle shows progressive deterioration. *Myotonic dystrophy* combines these two features—hence its name.

Less fortunately, doctors have used other names for myotonic dystrophy, which can confuse people; these are summarized in Table 1.1, but deserve a little explanation.

Table 1.1 Different names for myotonic dystrophy—and similar disorders

---

Other names for myotonic dystrophy
    Steinert's disease
    Myotonic muscular dystrophy
    Dystrophia myotonica
    Myotonia dystrophica
    Myotonia atrophica

Similar sounding names that are *not* myotonic dystrophy
    Muscular dystrophy (many other types)
    Myotonia congenita (Thomsen's disease)
    Congenital muscular dystrophy

In the past, doctors liked to use Latin names (to impress their patients?) so you may see the names *dystrophia myotonica*, *myotonia dystrophica*, or *myotonia atrophica*. They are just other names for myotonic dystrophy and it is best to avoid them. If you live in Continental Europe, you may have been given the name *Steinert's disease*. Steinert, a German doctor of the nineteenth century was one of the discoverers (see below), and Steinert's disease is no different from myotonic dystrophy. Altogether it is best to stick with the single name myotonic dystrophy. Where the disorder has begun at birth or in early childhood, doctors may use the terms *congenital myotonic dystrophy* or *childhood-onset myotonic dystrophy*.

Other *different* conditions with similar names include *myotonia congenita* (also called *Thomsen's disease*), in which there is no dystrophy and the muscles stay unchanged throughout life. The term *muscular dystrophy* refers to the whole group of disorders in which progressive weakness occurs in muscles, and this umbrella term includes myotonic dystrophy among many others. Most patients with muscular dystrophy will have other types, not myotonic dystrophy. It is especially important to know that *congenital muscular dystrophy* is *not* the same as congenital myotonic dystrophy (see Chapter 5).

What are the main problems?

Now that you are (hopefully) clearer about the name you have been given, it is time to outline the main features of myotonic dystrophy; later chapters go into them in more detail. Bear in mind that because myotonic dystrophy is so variable, these may not exactly match the problems you have recognized in yourself or your relative. However, if there is absolutely no similarity it is reasonable to question the diagnosis.

Table 1.2 lists some of the main problems found in adult patients with myotonic dystrophy, which lead them to seek medical help. Of course many people find it difficult to put their symptoms into precise words, so weakness may be expressed as 'tiredness' and the rather specific difficulty of relaxing muscles caused by myotonia is usually thought of as general stiffness, perhaps related to the joints rather than to the muscles.

The symptoms can be separated usefully into those due to the muscles themselves and those arising from other body systems. Since this second group can be as or more

Table 1.2 Myotonic dystrophy—the main symptoms in adults

Muscle symptoms
    Muscle weakness
    Muscular stiffness (myotonia)

Other symptoms
    Bowel disturbance and abdominal pain
    Disturbance of heart rhythm
    Daytime sleepiness
    Cataracts

important than the muscle symptoms it is most important to recognize from the onset that myotonic dystrophy is *not just a muscle disease*, it is a multi-systemic disease. Chapter 4 goes into these different symptoms in more detail.

At this point, it is important to emphasize how remarkably variable myotonic dystrophy is, not only in its severity but also in the type of symptoms and in the age at onset. In fact, it is probably the most variable disorder known in medicine, something that causes difficulties to doctors in recognizing it, as well as to patients and their families. Table 1.3 summarizes this, but it is important for anyone reading this book to recognize that not all of the problems described are likely to occur in a single person, that different members of a family may be very differently affected, and that some people with myotonic dystrophy, especially where it is recognized in later life, may never develop serious medical problems at all. Conversely, those with early onset, especially with problems from birth (congenital myotonic dystrophy), may show quite a different pattern of problems from those seen when onset is in adult life.

Inheritance is always a matter of importance and concern, once the diagnosis of myotonic dystrophy has been made and family members have recognized its genetic

Table 1.3 Myotonic dystrophy—a very variable condition

Age at onset	0–80 years
Severity of muscle problems	None to severe
Other types of problem	Can be absent, or may be more troublesome than muscle symptoms
Relationship to age at onset	In general symptoms more marked when onset earlier
Pattern in a family	Very variable, especially between generations

nature. Again, this is a topic important enough to deserve a separate chapter (Chapter 6), especially as many people have found it difficult to get access to accurate information on risks to relatives.

Our ability to answer questions about genetic risk and to undertake tests that will accurately show who in a family is or is not likely to develop myotonic dystrophy has been greatly advanced in the past few years. Genetic research has identified the actual gene involved and the change in it that results in this condition. This research has begun to help us understand how the genetic mutation causes changes in the muscles, heart, and other various organs, that can be affected. When one stops to think of the complexity of all these organs it is hardly

Table 1.4 Myotonic dystrophy—some landmarks

1909	First clear descriptions of myotonic dystrophy as a separate disorder (Steinert, Germany; Batten and Gibb, England)
1911	First association of myotonic dystrophy and cataract
1916	Detailed muscle changes analysed under microscope
1947	First full family and genetic studies
1960	Congenital form of myotonic dystrophy first recognized
1971	Initial mapping of the myotonic dystrophy gene
1992	Myotonic dystrophy gene identified
1994	First systematic therapy trials
2000	Myotonic dystrophy first reproduced in an experimental model
2001	Second gene, involved in a small number of patients, identified

surprising that unravelling all the different steps and interactions is proving a difficult, time-consuming (and costly) process; but compared with 10 years ago, our understanding has increased to an amazing extent, as I try to explain in Chapter 7.

Lastly in this opening chapter, come the questions that are the most important in everyone's minds. What can actually be done to help in terms of medical treatment, prevention, and cure? Or, if these are not possible at present, how can patients make sure they obtain the best available medical management, care, and general support? Here is where it has to be said that very much remains to be done, and I hope that writing this book will help, even if a little, to improve the situation. The last chapters of the book take up this theme.

For those people who like a historical approach, Table 1.4 gives some of the main landmarks in the recognition and understanding of myotonic dystrophy. It can be seen that almost a century has passed from the first description of the condition in 1909 but our understanding has probably progressed as much in the past 10 years as in the previous 90. Let us hope that this continues to be the case and that this increased understanding soon shows benefits in treatment.

I hope that anyone who has read this chapter, previously knowing nothing about myotonic dystrophy, will now at least feel a little familiar with the subject. Now it is important to take up the different topics in more detail.

2
Muscle symptoms and myotonic dystrophy

Making a diagnosis—and how the patient sees it

The first diagnosis of myotonic dystrophy in a patient may be made by a wide range of different doctors, depending on what type of symptom is initially most troublesome and leads the person to seek medical advice. Apart from specialists, an alert family doctor may suspect the condition; a paediatrician if the condition starts in childhood, or a clinical geneticist who has seen other family members, may be the first person involved—or you may recognize it yourself. But since most patients have muscle symptoms, it is the neurologist—a specialist in disorders of brain, nerves, and muscles—who will be involved in most cases, so it makes sense to start at this point and to look at the situation from the viewpoint of the person who has just consulted, or has just been referred to a neurologist, and outline the likely process of events—what can you expect to happen?

I have already indicated in the opening chapter that *weakness* and *stiffness* are the two main muscle symptoms that occur in myotonic dystrophy. For almost all patients it is weakness that is most troublesome, and you may find it irritating that doctors can appear to be more concerned by the stiffness (myotonia) than by the weakness.

However, in making a diagnosis of myotonic dystrophy it is the presence of *both* that is important; there are many causes of weakness and quite a number of causes of myotonia, but the finding of both together in a patient makes it almost certain that the diagnosis is myotonic dystrophy, even before any tests are done.

You may wonder at this point, if it is indeed so simple, why do so many patients with myotonic dystrophy not get diagnosed for many months or even years, and why are a significant number at first given the wrong diagnosis?

The answer to this is not entirely the fault or ignorance of doctors, since the diagnosis will only be made if it is in the doctor's mind; and this will depend not only on their knowledge, but on what symptoms are described. Even neurologists (apart from the few with a special interest) will only see a few myotonic dystrophy patients in a year, while doctors in other fields will only meet them rarely; so, unless the symptoms are clear, they are unlikely to be thinking about it. In fact, the symptoms are often vaguely expressed by patients (some even minimize or deny them); so with this combination all too often nobody considers the condition. I show some of the main reasons in Table 2.1.

Table 2.1 Reasons for myotonic dystrophy not being diagnosed

Doctor
  Not familiar with features
  Only rarely sees affected people
  Not listening to patient's story
  Not taking family history
Patient
  Not describing symptoms clearly
  Minimizing or denying muscle symptoms
  Not mentioning affected relatives

So, how can you be sure that you, or your relatives, avoid this unhappy situation? Table 2.1 provides some guidance; you can make sure you avoid the problems in the second part of the table, while with patience and persistence you should be able to ensure that doctors have the key information—especially if someone else in your family is already known to have the condition.

It is worth outlining at this point what are the particular features of muscle weakness that make a diagnosis of myotonic dystrophy and which help to rule out other forms of muscular dystrophy and other neurological conditions. First among these is the *pattern of muscle weakness* (see Table 2.2). This is very characteristic, especially the involvement of the face and jaw muscles, including drooping of the eyelids (medical term—ptosis) and weakness of the neck muscles, together with the small muscles of the hands and lower legs. Almost as important is the sparing of certain muscle groups, at least initially; these include especially the large muscles of thighs, shoulders, and trunk, which are often the first involved in other muscular dystrophies.

Myotonia, when present along with weakness, is very characteristic, which is why it is so important to mention any difficulty in relaxing muscles, especially grip, even if it does not bother you. Myotonia is tested for by asking a patient to first grip firmly, then let go rapidly, and also by firmly tapping the thumb muscles.

Some, though not many, myotonic dystrophy patients have troublesome stiffness from myotonia, but very little weakness. Here it can be difficult to distinguish other disorders where myotonia occurs but with no (or almost no) weakness, and which are quite distinct conditions with a very different outlook and inheritance. These other myotonic disorders are all very rare; the most frequent is termed *myotonia congenita* or Thomsen's disease.

Since many myotonic dystrophy patients have symptoms from other body systems, it is important that you

Table 2.2 Myotonic dystrophy—the muscle groups most affected

Muscle or muscle group involved	Medical name for muscles	Consequences for the affected person
Elevator of eyelids	Levator palpebrae	Drooping eyelids (Ptosis)
Facial muscles	—	Loss of expression
Jaw muscles	Temporalis; Masseters	Open jaw, mouth breathing (children especially); indistinct speech; jaw clicking or coming out of place
Neck muscles (especially forward movement)	Sternomastoids	Difficulty raising head; risk of 'whiplash' injury
Forearm and wrist muscles	Supinator; Wrist dorsiflexors	Difficulty lifting; Clumsiness
Small hand muscles	Interossei; Flexor pollicis	Difficulty with writing, fine movements (e.g. buttons); Stiffness (due to myotonia)
Lower leg muscles and ankles	Anterior tibial; Peroneal; Ankle dorsiflexion	Unsteadiness; Foot drop

mention these, even if they appear unconnected with the muscle problems. In fact, they can be very important indeed, as I show in the next chapter.

If you have a relative diagnosed with myotonic dystrophy—or with features suggestive of it—it is most important that you mention this information, even if not directly asked. This could save a lot of delay or difficulty, though of course it could turn out that your symptoms are quite unrelated. If you are able to get permission from your relatives for their records to be checked, then this will be even more helpful and may save tests being repeated on yourself.

All of the above steps can help to make sure that the diagnosis of myotonic dystrophy is strongly suspected (or alternatively made unlikely) after a single thorough consultation. It also means that any tests that are requested are more likely to be the right ones, rather than ones that will simply confuse things further.

The effects of muscle weakness

The characteristic pattern of muscle weakness is not only important to the doctor in making an accurate diagnosis; it also determines what the patient is unable, or finds it difficult to do, and so is the most important aspect of myotonic dystrophy as a muscle disease. Some of the main consequences of weakness of particular muscles are listed in Table 2.2; the anatomical names of the muscles are also given since these are often mentioned in medical records. You may recognize some of your own difficulties in this table, but it is again important to stress how variable myotonic dystrophy can be; for example, while for most patients getting out of a chair or standing alone (which requires the large anti-gravity muscles) is not an early problem, a few people show this prominently. Also you should bear in mind that a person's main symptoms will partly reflect their work or other activities and that the same degree of weakness will thus bother one person more than another.

There are many muscles that we do not think about at all—unless they go wrong. Thus the muscles involved in breathing and swallowing are vital, but any symptoms will not be thought of as muscle symptoms. This means that many of the general problems covered in the next chapter really have muscle weakness as the underlying cause, even though the patient (and the doctor) may not realize this.

Any muscle that is weak, whether from muscle disease, disuse, or because the nerve supplying it is disordered, will tend to waste; this is seen in most myotonic dystrophy patients to some extent and can be visible before symptoms are troublesome. Old photographs will often show the pattern of wasting and weakness, especially in the face; these can be very helpful to doctors in trying to date age at onset, or in deciding whether someone no longer living was affected.

Investigations

All the areas outlined above can form part of a medical consultation and do not require any special facilities and tests. It should be possible to make a firm diagnosis of myotonic dystrophy in the majority of cases at this point, providing that a careful history has been taken (including family history) and a thorough examination made. It will surprise many people to know that these are much more important than tests in making a diagnosis; if a doctor has missed the main features in the history and examination, then the wrong tests may be ordered and the results can be misleading.

Despite this, most patients will have some forms of test done, either to confirm the clinical diagnosis, or in situations where the findings on examination are very slight or not typical, and where other conditions need to be ruled out. Fortunately these are now fewer and less unpleasant than was the case a few years ago, thanks largely to the development of accurate genetic tests for myotonic dystrophy and other muscle disorders. Some further tests may be needed, not to make the diagnosis, but as part of management; these are dealt with later on in Chapter 9.

Tests can be conveniently divided into blood tests and muscle tests. Regarding blood tests, much the most important is the genetic test which looks for the particular change in the myotonic dystrophy gene, and which is present in almost all patients. This test is explained in more detail later from the viewpoint of family members, but it will confirm (or rule out) the diagnosis of myotonic dystrophy in most patients with symptoms thought to be due to the condition.

Another blood test measures the level of the muscle protein creatine kinase, which is raised in many muscle disorders and can give an indication of how active the condition is. A normal result does *not* mean a person does not have myotonic dystrophy.

There are two main types of muscle test: electrical tests and biopsy. Neither is pleasant, so careful thought should be given as to whether they are really needed. Electrical tests (electromyography (EMG)) will show the characteristic pattern of electrical discharge that is seen in true myotonia but not in other causes of muscle stiffness. When recorded on a loudspeaker it has a 'dive bomber' sound. A fine needle has to be placed in the muscle to record this and may be painful, but not very (I have had it done myself). Nowadays this test is mainly done when there are uncertainties or when no one else in the family has a definite diagnosis. However, the EMG is not absolute in its results. If the patient is minimally affected, myotonia might not show up on the test.

Muscle biopsy involves removing a piece of muscle for study down the microscope or by chemical analysis. This may need a small incision or it can be done with a (large) needle. Local anaesthetic should make it pain free, but it is not pleasant (I have had this done also!). Muscle biopsy does show rather characteristic changes in myotonic dystrophy, but it is now rarely an essential part of diagnosis. It may be very important to analyse muscle for research, but if this is the reason it is being done, you should be asked for your specific permission.

A note on two similar conditions that can be confused with myotonic dystrophy

Myotonia congenita (Thomsen's disease)

In this condition, as noted already, significant weakness does not occur, but the stiffness from myotonia is often much worse than in myotonic dystrophy. If you have this disorder, then this book is not written for you. Sadly, I cannot think of a suitable source of information, though the Internet may help. You may be interested to know that Dr Julius Thomsen, a Danish physician who described the condition some years before myotonic dystrophy was recognized, was himself affected. He published his description because his son, also affected, was in danger of being conscripted into the army because no one believed he had a medical condition.

Proximal myotonic myopathy

Proximal myotonic myopathy (PROMM—also sometimes termed type 2 myotonic dystrophy) is a recently recognized condition, which is closely related to myotonic dystrophy but has a different gene defect, which has now been specifically identified. It seems to be rare (except in Germany) and is best considered as a type of myotonic dystrophy, though the muscle weakness is more of the larger thigh (proximal) muscles. If you are one of the few people with PROMM, then probably much of this book will apply to you, but you should remember that the gene defect is different and that we are still beginning to learn about the range of features that it shows.

We have now reached the point where a firm diagnosis of myotonic dystrophy has been made and confirmed in yourself (or your relative). You will be wanting to know what this means for you and your family, and in particular, what the future will hold in terms of your muscle weakness. I try to cover this in the next chapter.

3
Looking ahead

How much worse will my muscle weakness get? And how rapidly? Will it spread to other muscles that are normal at present? Will I need a wheelchair later in life? Will I be more or less affected than my relatives?

Once a person has been diagnosed as having myotonic dystrophy and has accepted that they have a medical condition, these are some of the questions that arise and need answering. As you will see, they are not easy to answer, but it is possible to give at least a guide to a person's outlook. I shall deal here only with muscle symptoms; other effects on health are covered in the next chapter.

First, it is easy to deal with the outlook for muscle stiffness or myotonia—it rarely gets much worse after diagnosis and may in later years improve. But this is not of much help to patients since most people are little bothered by it anyway. It is the weakness that is the main concern. So what is the outlook for the weakness?

At this point, most doctors, especially those with a lot of experience of myotonic dystrophy like myself, will start to become rather cautious and imprecise, which you may find unhelpful. But the fact is that we know how very variable myotonic dystrophy can be, so if we are too precise in our prediction, we will very likely be wrong. It is best to go back to some of the questions and see how far they can be answered.

If you have myotonic dystrophy and already have significant muscle weakness, it will almost certainly get worse to some extent (unless an effective treatment is found). The extent of the worsening depends very much on your age; if you are already past 50 years and have only slight weakness, it may only increase slightly over the rest of your life. If you have no weakness at this age, but have been diagnosed by a genetic test or because of cataract, then you may never develop significant weakness at all. By contrast, if you have weakness develop in early adult life, it is likely to get worse steadily and can become severe after many years. However, if you have been diagnosed as a young person because of myotonia, not weakness, or because a relative is affected, then it is much less certain that weakness will also be a problem. Young children with the condition may improve for a period (see Chapter 5).

As to whether deterioration might be rapid, one can be very definite in saying that it will not. Myotonic dystrophy never changes suddenly (unlike, for example, multiple sclerosis), nor does it usually change its rate of progression. Thus the best guide is usually how much change there has been over the past 3, 5, or 10 years; one can project this into the future, at least approximately. Some people will change very little over a 5- or 10-year period, others more, but change is over years, not months. Many patients will undoubtedly outlast their doctors.

Most patients will never need a wheelchair, at least not for use in the house. This is because the large muscles needed for weight bearing and walking are usually only late and moderately affected. It is most important to recognize that myotonic dystrophy is completely different in this respect from Duchenne and similar muscular dystrophies. On the other hand, weakness of some other muscles may be a serious problem at a time when mobility is still reasonable.

It is very difficult to predict severity from what has happened in a relative; we now know that this is because the genetic change can itself vary within a family, ranging from minimal to severe in nature.

Does myotonic dystrophy shorten life? The simple answer is that it can, but not necessarily, and that many of the potentially fatal complications can be avoided. Most people with myotonic dystrophy do not die because of their muscle disease, but because of the more general problems that are covered in the next chapter, such as heart or lung problems or complications of surgery. Chapter 9 deals with how to avoid them and it is essential for you to recognize that most early deaths from myotonic dystrophy are preventable. If onset has been late in life, then lifespan is probably unaffected. Only in the severe congenital form is there a high mortality rate in the first months of life.

The conclusion is that as a newly diagnosed patient with myotonic dystrophy you should have many years of active and productive life ahead of you, provided that you take steps to know about your condition, look after yourself and avoid unnecessary problems, and have good medical care. A positive outlook on life will undoubtedly help you in this.

Patterns in a family

It is natural to assume that because someone else in the family has myotonic dystrophy in a severe form—or mildly—that you will follow much the same course. But this is often far from the case; one of the characteristic features of the disorder is how much it varies even within a single family. I shall explain why this is so in a later chapter. In general myotonic dystrophy shows more similarity between brothers and sisters (sibs) than it does between different generations. It often appears to be more severe in the younger than in the older generations and the contrast is especially seen in those severely affected children (see Chapter 5) whose mothers are often only mildly affected. The whole topic of genetic risks is dealt with fully in Chapter 6.

What can make things worse—or better?

At present there is no medical treatment that significantly alters the course of the condition, though a number of trials are getting underway. Nor are there clear-cut effects of diet and exercise (see Chapter 9). On the other hand there are a number of factors that can make your condition worse (Table 3.1), and since some of these can be avoided, it is as well to be aware of them.

Top of the list is injury, especially if this results in having a leg in plaster or being confined to bed for some weeks. It is surprising how much muscles can waste and become weaker simply by being out of action for a relatively short time. So you need to think carefully how you can avoid any injuries and if they do occur ensure you stay as mobile as possible.

Clearly some may be completely out of your control, and there is little point in shutting yourself away from all possible hazards, but many 'accidents' are really preventable, given some thought and planning. Look at your house: Are your stairs safe? Should you have rails, handles, or other aids (see Chapter 9) fitted? Perhaps you have put off having necessary things done? Or are you perhaps unwilling to admit that you have a problem? (too proud or stubborn are terms I have heard relatives use!).

Table 3.1 Factors that can make myotonic dystrophy worse

Injury
Immobility
Unplanned surgery or anaesthesia
Excess weight
Unawareness of (or ignoring) known complications
Being treated for wrong diagnosis

Conditions at work or driving are similar areas you will need to examine and you may need help with making changes, but the 'bottom line' is: *avoid injury at all costs.*

Immobility from illness or surgery is another reason why myotonic dystrophy can be made worse. In this situation the body often breaks down its own protein to use—and this includes muscle.

Weight is an important and difficult problem; being overweight probably does not actually alter the course of the disorder itself (though it can predispose to injury), but it certainly makes weakness seem worse—essentially you are asking already weak muscles to carry around an extra load, which is not sensible.

Pregnancy is probably not a significant aggravating factor, unless complications enforce immobility. It can certainly make a person increasingly tired, though, as can having to care for young children. Exercise is likewise probably not a harmful factor unless it makes injury more likely—but equally it is unlikely to improve the natural course of the weakness.

Altogether there are few 'do's and don'ts' that a person with myotonic dystrophy needs to follow except those which are common sense, as noted above. Nevertheless I have seen many people ignore these—and quite a few come to harm as a result—so I feel no need to apologize for emphasizing points that may seem obvious.

4

Not just a muscle disease

The wider effects of myotonic dystrophy

If you have just been diagnosed as having myotonic dystrophy, it is hard enough to accept having a muscle condition that might give serious problems in years ahead. To be told that in addition you might develop heart or other problems is a troublesome blow to patients, especially since the list of possible problems seems long and serious. I shall try in this chapter to put these aspects into a positive perspective and especially to show that recognizing the possibility and importance of these other aspects is of the greatest help in avoiding serious health problems, and is one of the main ways in which a person can plan positively and maintain control over their own health. Before this can happen, however, both patients and doctors have to accept that myotonic dystrophy is *not just a muscle disease*.

In Table 4.1 I list some of the main general health problems that may be associated with myotonic dystrophy. The list may appear alarmingly long, but I must stress that most patients have only some of the problems, that some have none of them and, most important, that some of the problems can be avoided, prevented, or treated by appropriate action, *if* they are recognized. As mentioned

Table 4.1 Myotonic dystrophy—general health problems

Heart	Disturbed rhythm
Chest	Frequent infections
Swallowing	Food sticking; choking
Bowel disturbance	Constipation, diarrhoea
Abdominal pain	Often associated with bowel disturbance
Poor vision	May be due to cataracts
Sleepiness	Especially daytime

earlier, some of these general problems are indirectly due to muscle weakness; others are the result of quite separate processes. Children with myotonic dystrophy often show rather different features and are considered in Chapter 5. Of course, myotonic dystrophy patients may develop completely separate disorders, so careful thought must be given to whether a particular symptom is related to myotonic dystrophy or not.

The heart

Since the heart is made of muscle, it is not too surprising that it may be affected in myotonic dystrophy. It should first be stressed that in many ways it is not. For example coronary heart disease (the commonest cause of death in many populations) is not increased, nor is high blood pressure or stroke. In fact, blood pressure is often low in myotonic dystrophy; this is harmless unless doctors make efforts to keep it 'normal' (for example, after surgery).

The main heart problem that may occur in myotonic dystrophy is disturbed conduction of the heartbeat. This results from small areas of heart muscle (the conducting tissue) being affected, often when the heart is otherwise normal. It can result in the heart rate being too fast, too slow, or irregular. Any of these disturbances can affect the heart's function and cause breathlessness, faintness, blackouts, or palpitations. Chest pain is less common. Any of these symptoms should be taken seriously and investigated, always including an electrocardiogram (ECG, EKG) and, depending on the situation, other heart investigations may be needed. If a heart specialist (cardiologist) or hospital physician (internist) is involved, then they must know you have myotonic dystrophy (they may not be familiar with it so it is worth giving them relevant information). If you have been under a neurologist, it is important that they do not forget the heart (which is not their own field of expertise).

Most heart conduction problems can be treated satisfactorily (see Chapter 9), but it is better if they can be prevented in the first place. Fortunately, the ECG provides a simple way of spotting likely problems ahead, especially if there is a slight slowing of conduction. For this reason it should be done on every patient when diagnosed and probably once a year thereafter. A normal ECG reduces (though not completely) the chance of any major heart conduction problem occurring in the near future, and it can be compared from year to year. It is important to recognize that heart disturbances can occur in patients whose muscle problems are relatively mild.

Chest and lungs

Although the lungs themselves are not directly affected in myotonic dystrophy, the breathing muscles (the diaphragm and intercostal muscles) are. This can cause problems in several ways. First, weak breathing muscles can make it difficult to cough and to clear secretions from the chest, resulting in repeated chest infections. This is a problem usually seen in more severely affected patients, but can be made worse if swallowing problems (see below) result in food 'going the wrong way' and entering the chest. If you have myotonic dystrophy and get chest infections, both the function of the breathing muscles and the possibility of swallowing problems should be looked into; special investigations may be needed for this.

The second problem that can result from weak breathing muscles is that oxygen levels in the blood drop, especially at night, causing drowsiness and headache; again these are aspects that need careful consideration. As with the ECG, so simple breathing tests on a regular basis may give an indication that problems could occur in future, while normal results make them unlikely.

Swallowing problems

Many myotonic dystrophy patients notice that their jaw and tongue may be stiff at times and cause difficulty in chewing and swallowing; sometimes the jaw can 'come out of place', but it usually returns on its own. This stiffness of chewing is probably due to myotonia in these muscles, but is less important than what happens in the 'involuntary' part of swallowing once food has left the mouth and travels down the gullet (oesophagus) to reach the stomach.

Here 'involuntary' or 'smooth' muscle is involved in the process and, if it is affected, as it may be in myotonic dystrophy, then food or liquids may stick at some point, or may enter the tubes leading to the lungs instead of the stomach. This can cause chest infections (see above), but also may make a person cough or splutter while eating or drinking; food may seem to stick and have to be washed down by drinking. If swallowing problems are significant, they may have to be investigated by special X-ray procedures, and much help can be obtained from the advice of a speech and swallowing therapist. Approaches to management are given in Chapter 9, but, as with heart problems, it is essential that patients and doctors recognize that they can occur as part of myotonic dystrophy.

Abdominal pain and bowel problems

These are extremely common in myotonic dystrophy and can be very troublesome to patients, though they are rarely dangerous in themselves. Their real danger is that surgeons or other doctors may misinterpret them and not realize that they are connected with myotonic dystrophy—or indeed that the patient has the condition at all. They only very rarely need surgical treatment, which can be dangerous and is unlikely to be of help.

Here is an excellent example of how important it is for all patients with myotonic dystrophy to be fully informed about the wider aspects of their condition, and to be prepared to inform their doctors when necessary.

Abdominal pain in myotonic dystrophy is usually colicky, often central, but variable in its location. It is probably due to uncoordinated contraction of the muscle in the wall of the large bowel, and is similar to the condition known as 'irritable bowel' or 'spastic colon'. It usually responds to drugs that relax bowel muscle (see Chapter 9), but can be severe in some people. Powerful painkillers are best avoided, as they can be addictive. A healthy, high-fibre diet is also a sensible measure. The pain can be mistaken for appendicitis, bowel obstruction, or gall-bladder inflammation, and can lead to surgery. Of course myotonic dystrophy patients are not immune from these serious problems, but you should never allow a surgeon to operate without knowing about myotonic dystrophy and its bowel problems; even then surgery is best avoided if possible, particularly as an emergency.

Variable diarrhoea and constipation can also be problems, with constipation a particular problem in affected children. These symptoms may need investigating to exclude other bowel diseases, such as bowel cancer, but again those doctors involved need to know about the diagnosis of myotonic dystrophy first.

Eye problems

Drooping eyelids have already been mentioned and are rarely a serious problem. Surgery can be done, but does not always give lasting help. A more important eye problem is cataract, which can occur at a relatively young age. The appearance of the early cataracts of myotonic dystrophy are rather characteristic, so eye doctors (ophthalmologists) may be the first to make the diagnosis. Fortunately the results of cataract removal are generally excellent and this procedure carries minimal risk since it can be done under very light or local anaesthetic.

For many years it has been known that some patients with myotonic dystrophy may have cataract as their only medical problem, with minimal or no muscle problems. This is especially seen in patients with onset in old age, who may not know they have myotonic dystrophy until a relative is diagnosed, on account of muscle symptoms. This was a complete puzzle until recently, but can now be explained in terms of the variability of the genetic change (see Chapter 7).

Although cataract is the main eye problem in myotonic dystrophy, various other disturbances can occur—the most frequent is excessive watering and irritation of the eyes—so it is always wise to have a complete eye assessment as part of the initial medical assessment, and for this to be repeated every few years, especially if there are signs of cataract. In the past, eye examination was used to detect those relatives who might develop the condition; this was not always accurate and has now been replaced by direct testing for the genetic change.

Sleepiness and related symptoms

Excessive sleepiness (somnolence) is a common complaint of myotonic dystrophy patients—and is often more noticed by their families. Many patients 'drop off to sleep' at the slightest opportunity, despite adequate sleep at night and not being particularly active all day. Although a variety of medications has been tried out, including modenafil, they are not always helpful, but many people are relieved to learn that it is a recognized part of the disorder. It is always important to rule out inadequate breathing as a cause (see above), but this rarely proves to be involved except in some severely affected patients.

Probably the excessive sleepiness arises from the brain, rather than the muscles, and some patients can show other features such as lack of energy or loss of initiative, which may have a brain origin. These problems are more frequent in childhood-onset disease. It needs to be stressed, though, that many myotonic dystrophy patients (probably the majority) do not have this type of problem and can be found successfully holding all types of responsible, often skilled, and professional jobs.

Hormone problems

These can occur in both men and women, and are probably under-recognized. Diabetes (very common in the general population) is probably somewhat increased in frequency, but is generally mild. Many more patients show a tendency to it on special tests, but most will not actually develop it.

Reduced fertility may occur in males, and results from atrophy of the testes. Impotence and other male sexual problems are almost certainly underestimated and may be increased, but, as with diabetes, it is difficult to know how much more frequent they are than in the population as a whole. Fertility is less reduced in women than in men, but in pregnancy a series of important problems may occur, which are dealt with in Chapter 6. Menstrual and other common gynaecological problems may also be increased in frequency.

Detailed investigation for these and other possible hormonal (endocrine) problems is probably not required for all patients, but only where there are suggestive symptoms or where simple tests (as for diabetes) suggest further action is needed.

I have not attempted to cover all the rare problems that can occasionally occur in myotonic dystrophy and which are not directly due to muscle disease. Perhaps the best course, if an apparently unrelated problem arises, is for you to ask your doctor to think carefully whether the problem might be related, especially before you are referred to a surgeon. If you do need investigation or treatment by a particular type of specialist, you should make sure that they do not forget 'the rest' of your condition. Remember—it is important to be informed so you can be your best advocate. Increasingly specialists are experts in a small area and may know very little outside this. Wherever possible you should be under the care of someone who is familiar with your condition *as a whole*, and who can coordinate the activities of different specialists. A well-informed family doctor is probably best placed for this, or a paediatrician for affected children. Best of all is a clinic especially for myotonic dystrophy patients and related disorders, but these are still few and far between. This is taken up again in Chapter 9.

Meanwhile the conclusion should be to know as much as possible about your condition and the possible problems that can arise. After reading this book, and having to live with your condition, you are likely to know more about it than most doctors do. Avoiding problems of general health is to a large extent, unlike the course of the muscle disease, in your own hands.

5
Children with myotonic dystrophy

So far in this book myotonic dystrophy has been considered as a disorder of adult life, and this is how most doctors and patients have perceived it until recently. Minor features can be found in some older children, if looked for, which usually would not have given problems until adulthood, but most patients with typical myotonic dystrophy are healthy as children.

However, there is an important group of patients, which is entirely different, where myotonic dystrophy can give serious problems in newborn babies or young children. Many of these problems are quite different from those of adults with myotonic dystrophy and they deserve a separate chapter. I have written it from the perspective of the parents of such a child, especially the mother, in contrast to the rest of the book where 'you' means the patient.

Let me start where most such parents start. You know nothing about myotonic dystrophy, there is no muscle disorder known in your family, but your newborn child has serious problems with breathing and feeding and may well be in an intensive care unit, even on a ventilator. Doctors have probably been uncertain initially as to what is the cause, but now they have diagnosed myotonic dystrophy. To make matters worse you, as mother, may have been found to have a mild degree of myotonic dystrophy, though you had considered yourself quite healthy. Now it appears you have passed this on to your child, but in a very severe form.

Anyone who has been in this position must inevitably feel that their life is in pieces, and a mixture of grief, guilt, and anger will probably mean that you take in very little of what is told to you initially. Reading this chapter is unlikely to help much either at first. But as time passes these feelings begin to change and you will begin to feel the need to know more about the blow that has struck your family, and if possible to do something. This is the time when it becomes important that you have accurate information about myotonic dystrophy and its effects on your child and yourself.

Very likely you may have already by now read something about myotonic dystrophy, but it may have told you little about children with it. Your baby's problems will seem quite different; you will have different questions and need different answers.

Let us start with the name—*congenital myotonic dystrophy*. 'Congenital' simply means present from birth, and this is the hallmark of congenital myotonic dystrophy, though in some infants the features at birth are slight or not recognized. In fact the condition may have started *before* birth and have given problems during pregnancy, which I shall come to later.

What are the main problems faced by a baby with congenital myotonic dystrophy? I list them in Table 5.1, but they all have a single underlying factor—the muscles are profoundly weak and underdeveloped.

Breathing problems are the most serious immediate hazard, and may mean that the baby needs transfer to intensive care. In the past many babies with this condition died at this point, partly because facilities for reviving them were less developed, but also because congenital myotonic dystrophy was not recognized—and many more babies died soon after birth anyway. The main cause of the breathing problems is that the breathing

Table 5.1 Congenital myotonic dystrophy—the main problems in a baby

Problem	Cause
Inadequate breathing	Poorly developed breathing muscles
Inability to feed or suck	Weak swallowing and face muscles
Little or no facial movement	Face muscles especially weak
Floppiness; little spontaneous movement	Muscles generally weak and immature
Feet downturned ('talipes')	Imbalance of muscles in the womb

muscles are very weak and poorly developed; an added problem is that healthy babies 'breathe' in the womb, which helps both to develop the muscles and to mature the lungs. Babies with myotonic dystrophy have weak breathing muscles and stiff lungs to inflate as well—the combination may mean that the baby cannot survive.

Swallowing and feeding are the next hurdle a baby faces; again this requires well-developed and coordinated muscles and in congenital myotonic dystrophy these are the very ones (face, jaw, palate) that may be the most affected. As in adults, food may enter the lungs and cause chest problems even in a baby who has initially been able to breathe normally. Special feeding bottles as used for premature babies may be helpful.

Many babies with the condition move very little and when lifted they appear floppy (medical term—hypotonic). You may have noticed as mother that your baby moved very little in the womb also. This general lack of movement reflects the fact that most muscles of the body are weak and poorly developed; under the microscope it appears as if they have become arrested at an early stage of fetal life.

This generally poor muscle development may have a number of consequences that at first seem unconnected with muscle disease. For example, the feet may be down-turned and in a fixed position, known as 'talipes'. Sometimes there may be other joint contractures too. This again reflects the fact that the baby has not been moving normally in the womb and that imbalance of different muscle groups produces a fixed position.

I have already mentioned that many mothers of such affected children have already noticed problems in later pregnancy, such as lack of movement. Sensitive ultrasound scans can often now pick up abnormal joint positions. A further problem in pregnancy may have been excessive fluid in the womb (medical term—hydramnios or polyhydramnios). This probably results from the baby failing to swallow the fluid that surrounds it, which then builds up.

All in all I have painted a very serious picture of congenital myotonic dystrophy—and it is indeed a serious condition for babies who have the combination of problems that I have outlined—and which you may yourself have experienced at first hand. Despite all efforts and the facilities of modern neonatal intensive care, many babies still die, while the outlook for those who survive is also far from good. In general, the more serious the initial problems and the longer a baby requires to be supported by artificial ventilation, the greater is the chance that they will not survive.

I shall come to the problems in later childhood and adult life of patients with congenital myotonic dystrophy, but one question often has to be faced at this early stage by both parents and doctors: how far should one go and how long should one persist with active treatment such as artificial ventilation? There is no easy answer to this and indeed it is right that such decisions should not be easy, but I personally feel that it is important that all parents finding themselves in this situation should be involved in decision-making, together with their doctors. Whatever decision is made will depend partly on the severity of the illness at the time in the particular infant and partly also on the personal wishes and ethical or religious views of yourselves as parents. Another important factor should also be knowledge of what are the likely outcome and problems of the condition, long term as well as immediate. It is difficult for parents who know little or nothing of the disease, and who are inevitably distressed by what has happened, to make a fully informed decision, on which may hang profound long-term consequences. However, whatever your decision is, it should be accepted and supported by all the professionals involved.

Diagnosing congenital myotonic dystrophy

How can you be sure that your child really does have myotonic dystrophy, rather than one of the numerous other serious disorders of muscle and nerve that can affect newborn babies? The answer is that it may be far from easy, which accounts for why diagnosis is often delayed. Fortunately this has improved, partly because more paediatricians, especially those dealing with newborns, are aware of the condition and partly because genetic testing on blood will show not just the specific change of myotonic dystrophy, but also that the change is extremely large, characteristic of this severe form. The third reason, more worrying, is that you yourself, as mother, will probably have been found to have minor signs of the condition, even though you yourself may not have realized it. A family history of myotonic dystrophy in other branches of the family may also have given the clue, but the finding of myotonia and perhaps some slight weakness in you, together with the combination of problems in your baby, will have led to genetic testing and confirmed that myotonic dystrophy is indeed the problem.

These wider family issues are taken up in the next chapter.

The next few years

If your baby has survived the serious problems of the first weeks of life, or if the condition has not been so severe at this stage, what can you expect during the next few years of childhood? First, and very important, it is most unlikely that your baby will die during this time, unless there are serious remaining problems from a long period of intensive care. In fact things are likely to improve in terms of breathing and feeding, though these may remain problem areas. The normal 'milestones' of sitting and walking will almost certainly be slow, but they will be reached in time; foot problems may need physiotherapy or occasionally surgery, but your child will definitely walk and be able to walk unaided. This is quite unlike some other muscle disorders of infancy, so it is most important that you and those professionally involved realize this; an active approach is needed and you should not be deterred by being told that your child will never walk—he or she will, in time.

The floppiness of the newborn period also gradually disappears, but some degree of stiffness (myotonia) may appear in its place, though it is rarely significant. (If a baby or young child has marked myotonia, it is most unlikely to be due to myotonic dystrophy but rather one of the other myotonic disorders, and the diagnosis should be questioned.)

A number of physical problems are likely to remain though, and can become more marked; sometimes the diagnosis is only recognized at this point. The weakness of the face muscles can be very conspicuous, as is the weak jaw; these can make speech indistinct, and the lack of expression can be mistaken for lack of understanding.

A major issue that now starts to arise is that of intellectual development, and this is likely to be of equal or more concern to parents than physical problems. Unfortunately, in contrast to adult onset myotonic dystrophy, most children with congenital onset will indeed have significant intellectual impairment, something which seems to be present from birth or before, and which is often reflected in changes seen on a brain scan. It does not normally deteriorate and it varies greatly between children; it is not wholly the result of breathing problems at birth and it is often difficult to assess accurately due to muscular speech difficulties and lack of facial expression. But in general it is a serious problem in its own right, and its consequences have especially to be faced as questions of education and later life begin to be considered.

Understandably many parents are reluctant to accept that their child may have this extra burden on top of serious physical problems. But it is important to accept it, at least as a possibility, and to make sure that detailed physical and psychological assessments are obtained at an early stage to sort out as far as is possible how much of a child's developmental delay is due to physical and how much to mental problems.

Adolescence and beyond

Our long-term knowledge of children born with congenital myotonic dystrophy is limited by the fact that it has not long been widely recognized. Also many of those born 30 years ago who died would now have survived into adult life. So what we do know has to be viewed as provisional.

Again only few will die in later childhood, adolescence, or early adult life, so as a parent you must prepare for the long term. As with other healthy families, it is likely that you may die before your child. In terms of physical health, the more typical 'adult' features of myotonic dystrophy begin to develop in later childhood and become more conspicuous in adolescence. Adults will generally show more severe than average muscle disease, but it does not seem to deteriorate more rapidly than in adult-onset patients. It is very important that medical contact is not lost when a patient leaves the paediatric age group; this is where a specialist muscle clinic can help to ensure continuity. The general health problems involving swallowing and bowels can be troublesome, especially constipation, which can lead to a build up of faecal material. It is important to mention also that the anal muscles can be very lax, leading to soiling; also this can be misinterpreted by doctors as being due to sexual abuse. I have seen this cause great distress to a family and doctors must be aware that there is a direct link with the constipation and bowel muscle deterioration that occurs in the anal region, as elsewhere. A regular electrocardiogram (ECG) to monitor heart conduction is most important, as with adults.

Most difficult for parents to face are the consequences of mental impairment. A study by my colleagues and myself has shown that very few patients with congenital onset achieve an independent life or are able to hold a job unaided. This is probably the result of combined mental and physical disability, but it imposes a severe long-term burden on families; it also means that very careful thought and planning, with as much help as possible from local authorities, schools, and other agencies, is required if as satisfactory a long-term outcome as possible is to be reached.

Finally, what about the rest of the family? You, as mother, are likely to have myotonic dystrophy yourself. When your baby was born, this may have been insignificant, but even so it is essential that you take the precautions over surgery and other aspects described in other parts of this book. By the time your child is 20 years old, you may well have some significant problems yourself, and you should make sure you are checked and monitored regularly as a patient, rather than just attending clinic as a mother. Avoid physical tasks like heavy lifting and in general look after yourself, rather than let your life revolve round your affected child. After all, you are more than specially needed and you owe it to yourself and your family to remain as well as possible.

If you have other children, they may or may not also be affected, whether boys or girls. The question of genetic risks is covered in Chapter 6 and it is important that you as patient and parent should have full and accurate information on the chances of myotonic dystrophy occurring again in your family.

Myotonic dystrophy with childhood onset

This forms a group part way between those with onset at birth (congenital myotonic dystrophy) and those with adult onset disease. These children do not have the severe medical problems around birth seen in the congenital form and either father or mother can be the parent affected. Usually, it is problems of mental development or behaviour that are most prominent; muscle symptoms may not be noticed for some time, until it becomes clear that the child indeed has physical as well as intellectual difficulties. It is most important that schools and others involved appreciate this combination; serious medical problems in childhood are normally few, but the importance of monitoring medical aspects, such as the heart, and taking precautions related to surgery, must be emphasized.

6
Family aspects and genetic risks

So far in this book we have looked at myotonic dystrophy from the viewpoint of the affected person and their problems—the diagnosis, the pattern and course of the disorder, the wider effects, and the particular issues concerning affected children. But at an early stage of being investigated medically, you will have probably heard the terms 'genetic' and 'hereditary'; questions may have been asked about your family by doctors that give the impression that they are expected to be affected even if they are not. It is possible that you already know of relatives with myotonic dystrophy or something that sounds like it; or, most worrying, you may connect problems in your children, or other close relatives, with your own diagnosis.

This is a heavy burden, and we have touched on it already when considering severely affected children and their mothers. But it borders on many sensitive areas: families are all very different to each other and different branches may not always get on well together. Some families are scattered all over the world and may have little or no contact. 'Children' rapidly become grown up and need to make their own decisions in life, while grandparents may be old and frail, and reluctant to accept that a condition may be running in the family. Altogether there are lots of difficulties that need to be considered.

This chapter is also written for the relative who, while healthy themselves, may have just learned that myotonic dystrophy has been diagnosed in the family. What risks does this information—often coming out of the blue— have for you in this position, and for your own family?

Some people at this point shut their eyes to the possibility of these wider family risks and bury the whole subject. This is quite understandable, but it is unwise, partly because real harm may result from ignorance, partly because the true situation will usually emerge sooner or later, and relatives may feel angry and bitter that they have not been given important information. Most importantly, professional help is now available that can ease the burden and can help to answer the questions that relatives will have which you are unable to answer fully yourself.

Having worked as a medical geneticist—a doctor whose specialty is inherited disorders and their risks—for over 30 years, dealing with a wide range of conditions besides myotonic dystrophy, I have experienced at first hand most of the questions and many of the difficulties that arise, and I shall try to outline the main ones in this chapter. I have generally found that even when one cannot give as accurate answers to questions as one would like, or when the answers may seem discouraging, most people find it helpful to have had the chance to ask their questions and the time to go over their concerns in detail.

A word about inheritance

Myotonic dystrophy is indeed a disorder that results from a genetic alteration and which can be inherited, so it is important to know how it is inherited before going into the practical aspects of genetic risks.

The working of our bodies is at least partly determined by genetic factors or genes (around 30 000 of them altogether). If any of these goes wrong in some way, an inherited disorder can result. In myotonic dystrophy just one specific gene is altered (the details are covered in Chapter 7); this gene has now been identified and the alteration causing myotonic dystrophy can be detected by a genetic test.

Each of us has two copies of every gene (one from each parent). For some genetic disorders (including myotonic dystrophy), only one of these two copies needs to be altered to cause the disorder. This means that every affected person has both an altered and a normal copy.

You may find the simple diagram and family tree (Fig. 6.1) helpful in understanding this and following how the condition can be handed on. I have shown parents and two children as an example. Note that in family trees males are represented by a square and females by a circle.

In the example it is the father who is affected with myotonic dystrophy, but you can see that he also has a normal copy of the gene. When a child is conceived only one of the two copies of any gene will be passed on, the child's second copy coming from the other parent, who will almost always have two normal copies. So whether a child will inherit myotonic dystrophy depends on which copy is passed on by the affected parent; since either is equally likely, the chance is 50% or 50:50 (see Table 6.1).

I have shown the daughter inheriting the condition, but it is equally likely for males and females to inherit— or to transmit it. I hope that this example will have explained the 50% risk which is the basis for many of the genetic risks in myotonic dystrophy.

If we look at the figure again and imagine that the son and daughter are now asking about risks for their own children, then we can clearly see that there is no risk for children of the son, since both his copies of the gene are normal. However the daughter has the same 50% risk for her own children as was present in the previous generation.

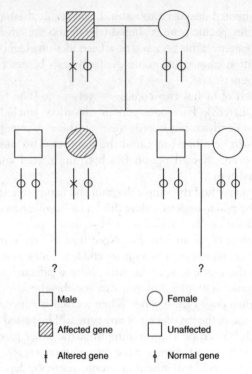

Figure 6.1 Genetic risks in myotonic dystrophy

This very simple pattern, known as *autosomal dominant* inheritance, holds universally for myotonic dystrophy families and all of the uncertainties described below are not because the inheritance of the altered gene varies, but rather because the way in which the alteration

Table 6.1 Genetic risks in myotonic dystrophy

Offspring of affected parent	50%
Offspring of definitely unaffected parent	0

actually shows itself as myotonic dystrophy can vary considerably.

Before leaving the simple pattern, it is important to correct some wrong ideas relating to the 50% risk that can arise. I have met the following.

1. I have two children and they both have myotonic dystrophy. How can this happen when you said the risk was 50%?

2. I have just had a child with myotonic dystrophy. Since the chance was 50%, does this mean I can go ahead and have another without the risk of it being affected?

3. I was the first born in my family and inherited the condition. Will my own first child be at particular risk?

The answer to all these three questions and others like them (see Table 6.2) is that the 50% risk applies *each time* a child is conceived; there is no link between one child being affected and the risk for others, nor is there any effect of order. It is no different from the chances of a coin thrown in the air landing head or tail uppermost.

Now we can move on to some of the other questions you will have about inheritance.

Table 6.2 Genetic risks in myotonic dystrophy

Factors *not* involved in size of risk
Birth order in family
Male or female (parent or offspring)*
Whether previous child affected or not
Number of other affected people in family
Severity of disease in parent*

*These factors can be involved in severity of disease (see text), though they do not affect size of risk.

Children born to an affected parent

I have already explained that such children have a 50% chance of *not* inheriting the condition, regardless of whether the affected parent is male or female, or mild or severely affected. But for a child that has inherited the altered gene these factors do influence the likely age at onset and severity. Here the estimates become much less clear cut, and I have not given actual figures here, but you will benefit from expert genetic counselling.

In general any offspring of an affected parent is somewhat more likely to have the disorder at earlier onset and more severely than in their parent, though this is on average, and not always the case. Why this is so is explained in the next chapter, but basically the genetic change is unstable and can increase from generation to generation. This is called 'anticipation'.

Secondly, affected women have a significant risk of having an affected child with the severe congenital form, while this only exceptionally occurs when the father is the affected parent. The reason underlying this difference seems to be that sperm carrying the very large genetic change causing the congenital form either do not survive or are not able to cause fertilization. It should be noted that only women who are symptomatic (often very mildly) are at high risk for a child with congenital myotonic dystrophy, but if such a child has already been born then it is likely that any other *affected* child will also have severe disease. (This also means that apparently unaffected children of such a woman will be more likely *not* to have inherited the condition.)

Risks for healthy relatives

Once myotonic dystrophy has been diagnosed in a family, it will not be long before other, apparently healthy relatives, begin to ask whether they themselves or their own children might be at risk for developing the disorder, or of passing it on. The extent and rate to which this enquiry happens will vary greatly between families and it is natural that this is so. Some members will take time to come to terms with the possibility of risk, while others will wish to have answers as soon as possible. Here again is where professional help in genetic counselling from a medical genetics service will be needed. It is important to avoid the situation where a large number of relatives are all worried, have conflicting views on what needs to be done, and do not know where to turn for help. So, if you are a close relative of someone who has been diagnosed with myotonic dystrophy, say a brother or sister, how can you obtain the advice and help you need? Here are some suggestions.

First you should ask yourself whether you have noticed any symptoms that could be due to myotonic dystrophy. Clearly muscle weakness or stiffness could be relevant, but so could early cataract or unexplained heart irregularity. It could be that you have already been worrying about such symptoms for years but have not sought medical advice, or that doctors have not found or thought of myotonic dystrophy as a possibility. If you are in this position, then being recognized as having myotonic dystrophy may come as a relief, and it will certainly help to avoid potentially serious medical hazards. The right course for you will be to seek expert medical advice, be thoroughly examined, and to leave genetic questions until it is clearer whether you are actually affected or not.

But if you are quite healthy, or if your imagined symptoms turn out to be nothing to do with myotonic dystrophy, there will still be questions along the lines of might I still develop the condition later? Or, even if I stay healthy might I pass it on? Here we come back to genetic counselling and it is likely that a specialist in this will be more familiar with handling these issues than most busy neurologists or physicians, whose main concern, understandably, is with those who actually have a medical disorder.

It may be helpful if I describe my own practice in this situation, as a guide to what may happen. First I take a careful history, asking particularly about symptoms that might relate to mild or early myotonic dystrophy, followed by a family history, with as much detail as possible on affected members. Next comes a physical examination, looking for mild weakness or myotonia that might not have caused any symptoms. Finally, I try to put things together and explain them to the person being seen.

What may the outcomes be? First, definite abnormalities may be present, even though they have not been noticed; this happens surprisingly frequently, though in some cases I suspect a person has chosen not to notice them.

Secondly, there may be some suspicious features present, but not enough to be sure. Here I usually tell a person that this is the situation, and that tests may be needed to be sure one way or another.

Thirdly (and most often), there is nothing abnormal to find on either history or examination—in other words you do not have myotonic dystrophy *now*. This is usually a great relief, but it does not answer the question as to whether it might develop in future. This is where genetic tests can help, as explained later.

In fact one can give a reasonably good indication of the future without any tests at all. Several studies have shown that around 90% of adults with an affected parent or sib and who are normal on clinical assessment will turn out to have a normal genetic test result; in other words myotonic dystrophy usually shows itself by early adult life if carefully looked for. Also if it does develop in later life it tends to be mild, so a completely healthy adult relative can be reassured about their own future health to a considerable extent.

But what if your main worries are about passing the condition on, either to your existing family or to any future children you may have? Only a genetic test can answer this with certainty, and fortunately such tests are now possible, accurate, and widely available. Before having a genetic test, however, you should think carefully about what your main question is. Is it whether you yourself have myotonic dystrophy at present? If so it is careful medical examination you need, followed up by further medical investigation if there are definite or suspicious signs present. If your questions are mainly about inheritance, then a genetic test will be more helpful. Basically, medical queries need medical answers; genetic queries need a genetic approach. Of course many, perhaps most people will be helped by a combination of both.

Genetic tests for myotonic dystrophy

This is an area that has developed radically over the past 10 years, as a result of research identifying the genetic change that causes myotonic dystrophy, described in the next chapter. Prior to this, older tests used markers close to the gene, or eye or muscle tests that may show early changes before symptoms develop. Anyone who was told that they would or would not develop myotonic dystrophy based on these older tests should remember that they had a definite margin of error. Since 1993 most genetic tests have been specific for the altered gene and are highly accurate (though no test is infallible).

The genetic alteration causing myotonic dystrophy is present in a person throughout their life, from conception to death, regardless of whether or not they have developed symptoms. This is quite unlike most medical tests, which are only abnormal when someone actually has the condition concerned, or perhaps is on the point of developing it. It is most important that anyone having a genetic test for myotonic dystrophy, especially if they are symptom free, understands that having the genetic abnormality is *not* the same as having the disorder.

Table 6.3 Genetic testing for myotonic dystrophy

Diagnostic	Helps to tell whether myotonic dystrophy is the cause in a person with symptoms suggesting it
Presymptomatic (predictive)	Indicates whether a healthy relative is likely to develop or pass on the disorder
Prenatal	Will tell whether or not a pregnancy has inherited the condition
Preimplantation	Indicates whether an embryo has inherited the condition before it is implanted in the womb

Genetic tests in myotonic dystrophy can be used in several very different situations, and even though the laboratory aspects of the test are similar in all of them, the wider aspects are not. Table 6.3 summarizes their main use.

Diagnostic genetic testing is extremely useful in patients with symptoms where myotonic dystrophy is likely or a possibility. Because the test, usually on blood, is very specific (it is not abnormal in other types of muscle disease) and sensitive (virtually all myotonic dystrophy patients worldwide show the change), it has become the main method of confirming the diagnosis and has largely replaced such tests as muscle biopsy and electrical tests, except in special situations. It can also be used when there is no known family history. As already mentioned, the genetic alteration varies in extent and to some degree this relates to severity and age at onset. Congenitally affected children show the largest changes; while patients with only cataract show the smallest, but in between there is only a very loose relationship with the course of the disorder, so the test result is not a reliable guide to outlook in a single individual. As a way of confirming or ruling out myotonic dystrophy, however, it is highly accurate. The recently recognized and much rarer 'type 2' mutation is dealt with in the next chapter.

Presymptomatic testing

I have already said that the genetic test will detect the gene alteration of myotonic dystrophy regardless of whether a person has symptoms or not and so can greatly help those healthy relatives who wish to be certain whether they might carry the alteration and so possibly pass it on or develop problems themselves later. Genetic testing for healthy people at risk for late-onset disorders overall has raised a lot of important issues, and is something quite new in medical practice. In general a specialist in medical genetics will be best placed to undertake this type of testing and to go through the complex and sometimes difficult issues involved. This is unlike diagnostic testing for people with symptoms, which is generally requested by neurologists and other disease specialists.

It is most important that before you, as a healthy person at risk, have presymptomatic testing for myotonic dystrophy, you have the test and its consequences fully explained, and that you have adequate time to think through whether you really want it or not. The test should *never* be done casually, as a matter of routine, just because the doctor thinks it is a good idea, or because others in the family feel you should have it. It is an important decision and it should be yours to make. Written consent for it should be given—but this is no substitute for full explanation and information.

Of course, the main reason people request a presymptomatic test is that they hope to be shown *not* to carry the genetic change, in which case they can be reassured that they are most unlikely to develop myotonic dystrophy or to pass it on. But you must remember that you could receive an abnormal result (though the odds as a healthy adult are in your favour as noted above) and you must be prepared for this in advance, not simply trust to chance that your result will turn out all right.

Here are some of the points you will need to think through.

1. Are you familiar enough with the condition, its full range of severity, and its effects? (Some people may not have this as personal experience if they do not have a close living affected relative.)

2. Are you prepared to live with knowing that you definitely have inherited the genetic change, rather than this just being a possibility?

3. Could there be consequences for work or insurance of having an abnormal test result?

4. What will the reaction of your family be to the result?

5. Will you tell your children that they themselves are now at 50% risk as a consequence of your result?

6. If you are planning to have more children, would you wish to have tests in pregnancy?

You can see that all these are issues that need much thought—before testing, not after. Making a decision may be difficult and you need both information and the time to process it. This is where a genetic counselling service can be of real help, since genetics specialists are familiar with the range of issues and can help you think through them, without putting you under pressure one way or the other. It is very rare for neurologists or comparable clinicians to have the experience or time to do this thoroughly, which is why I am in no doubt that presymptomatic genetic testing should normally be done by a medical genetics service. Regardless of who undertakes it, you should make sure that all the issues are gone through thoroughly and with adequate time. If the doctor you are seeing is not prepared to do this, you should ask to be referred to one who is.

Testing children

This is a difficult area that needs careful thought. As with all aspects of genetic testing, the rule should be think first, test later—not the other way around! If a baby or young child is thought by a paediatrician or child neurologist possibly to have myotonic dystrophy, then genetic testing can be very helpful; the test will either confirm the clinical diagnosis or rule it out, as with adults. But testing of *healthy* children with a family history of myotonic dystrophy is a different matter.

I have already indicated that for a healthy adult, deciding about testing needs very careful thought; not all people conclude that they wish to be tested. Young children cannot make these decisions or give consent, so unless there is a special medical indication, most professionals feel it is wise *not* to test young children but to wait until they are older and can make their own decision, or at least take part in it. Parents generally agree with this approach, once the issues have been carefully discussed. But sometimes parents feel they have the duty—and the right—to have their young children tested, regardless of what professionals advise. In my own experience this only happens very rarely, and I do not think that there should be a rigid rule against testing young children, but I do feel that it should be exceptional and that parents should have time to consider the issues before any testing is arranged. Usually parents are concerned mainly about their child's health, and a careful examination will give reassurance on this. Genetic tests are needed mainly for genetic decisions, which become relevant when the child is older. It should go without saying that no doctor should advise genetic testing on a healthy child simply because it is technically possible.

Adolescents requesting testing are a rather different scenario from young children. Many will really want to know if they are healthy, which is best answered by a careful physical examination. If a young person wishes to have a genetic test and has had the chance to discuss the issues fully (preferably on their own), then I see no reason not to go ahead; quite often such people are satisfied by having had the chance to discuss the family disorder with a genetic counselling expert and decide to leave testing until later.

Grandparents and other older relatives

It is common for a person diagnosed with myotonic dystrophy in adult life, perhaps already with an affected child, not to have either of their own parents known to be affected. We now know though that almost always the genetic change will have been passed on by one or other of the older generation; deciding whether to do anything about this or how to go about it requires a lot of tact and consideration.

Because of the tendency for myotonic dystrophy to occur earlier in successive generations, grandparents will commonly be mildy affected; often with cataract alone and no muscle disease of any significance. Some may be normal in every way and yet still carry the genetic change in a minor form. Such people will understandably feel upset and often guilty from the realization that they may themselves have passed on a condition that has given serious problems for their children and possibly been fatal in a grandchild.

Sometimes grandparents are asked to provide a blood sample for family investigation without having the opportunity to think about the implications or even to have an explanation of why it is important. This should not happen, and if such testing is to be done, then these older members should receive the same careful consideration as their younger relatives. It is quite possible that grandparents may prefer not to be tested, especially if neither has any symptoms.

For those older people who are tested, one can usually be confident that their own health is not likely to be significantly affected, especially if the genetic change is found to be minimal in extent. It is important that they realize this. Equally, if mild features of muscle disease are present but have not been recognized, then knowing that myotonic dystrophy is present in a mild form should be helpful in avoiding problems from anaesthesia or surgery.

Testing in pregnancy

The genetic test can detect whether a pregnancy has inherited the alteration for myotonic dystrophy and this can be done in early pregnancy so those who wish to have children but not to pass on the disorder can have termination of pregnancy if their own ethical and religious views and the laws of their country permit this. As with presymptomatic testing, this is a very personal and individual decision and not one that should be influenced by the views of doctors or other professionals.

Actually, only a few people do request prenatal testing and these are mostly couples where a child with severe congenital myotonic dystrophy has been born in the family. Since all tests in pregnancy carry some risk of causing miscarriage, it is not considered wise to undertake this when termination would not be wished for if the result proves abnormal.

Prenatal testing for myotonic dystrophy is best carried out at around 10 weeks of pregnancy, using the procedure known as chorion villus sampling (CVS), in which a piece of membrane around the embryo is removed using a needle, either through the abdomen or through the vagina. A result usually takes 1–2 weeks. Later testing can be done at around 15 weeks by the procedure of amniocentesis, where a fluid sample is removed from the womb, but here the cells in the fluid have to be grown in tissue culture, which can take an extra 2–3 weeks.

Wherever possible, if you wish to have prenatal testing you should plan ahead and discuss the issues fully with a genetic counselling professional, *before you become pregnant*. This will give you a contact person for when you are pregnant, who knows about you, and about myotonic dystrophy, already. Once you are indeed pregnant and have decided you want testing, you should inform your contact *at once*, since arranging tests with the laboratory and gynaecologist can take time. Do not wait to be referred to an antenatal clinic, and do not expect your obstetrician/gynaecologist to know much about myotonic dystrophy unless there has been a chance for previous discussion.

Since most women requesting prenatal tests are themselves affected with myotonic dystrophy, it is very important that you as mother are not forgotten in the process. There are several important problems that can occur which affect you, mainly in later pregnancy or around delivery. Table 6.4 lists some of these; make sure your obstetrician is aware of them and prepared. These problems can happen even if your baby does not have the condition. If there is a chance that your baby might have congenital myotonic dystrophy, then this must also be prepared for and an experienced paediatrician informed

Table 6.4 Risks in pregnancy for mothers with myotonic dystrophy

Excess fluid in the womb—'hydramnios'
Rapid delivery
Excessive bleeding after delivery
Risks of anaesthesia and surgery if caesarean section needed
Depressed breathing if heavy sedation needed

well in advance. Of course, if it is your partner, not your-self, who is affected, then one would not expect any special problems with pregnancy or delivery.

All of this means that any pregnant mother with myotonic dystrophy, especially if the baby could be severely affected, should receive antenatal care and deliv-ery in a hospital unit with full facilities, and with full back up for care of both mother and baby after delivery, should problems occur.

Pre-implantation genetic diagnosis

Pre-implantation genetic diagnosis (PGD) is just begin-ning to become possible, but is still at an early stage. Essentially, what is done is to mix egg and sperm outside the womb (*in vitro* fertilization, IVF) and then test sev-eral embryos in the hope that at least one does *not* show the genetic change and can then be placed in the womb. This gives the option of avoiding termination of preg-nancy, but it has to be remembered that the IVF proce-dure itself is complex and has a low success rate (around 20% each time) and that it is not generally available as part of free health care. This could change in the near future. The laboratory aspects are also extremely tricky and at present (end of 2001) I know of only one centre in the world (in Brussels) with adequate published expe-rience, where I would be happy to refer a patient. There are several others at an early stage and (unfortunately) also a number of centres making unwarranted claims. If you are considering PGD as an option you should first be seen for genetic counselling and then ask the geneticist involved to obtain full information about what centres exist and what they can (and cannot) do. It is unwise to ask for direct referral to a PGD centre yourself, since there may be many aspects that need sorting out first.

I hope that in this chapter I have covered most of the difficult questions which you and your relatives will wish to ask about family and genetic issues. Sadly, they are often still given less attention by doctors than the medical aspects of myotonic dystrophy. If you feel this is the case with yourself, then you should ask for referral to a genetic counselling clinic, where you should be given time and freedom to bring up the issues important to you without being under pressure. Increasingly, most neurologists also recognize the value of this too, and that, apart from those with special experience, they are not best placed to handle the queries of healthy family members. A close link and partnership exists between the specialties of neurology and genetics in most regions, and in most countries there is a network of genetic clinics that can help to ensure that you no longer have to carry the worry and burden of the family aspects unaided.

7
Advances in research

What do we really know about the causes of myotonic dystrophy?

So far I have said very little about research, but have concentrated on the practical aspects of diagnosing the disorder, its clinical problems involving muscle and other body systems, and the particular areas of childhood disease and the genetic aspects. Most people will be more concerned with the long-term aims of research—effective treatment and prevention of symptoms—than with the details of the research itself. But you will want to have a picture of how things stand at present; which areas are advancing rapidly and may give clues to treatment; and also whether you can help in any way. I shall try to summarize things in a simple manner in this chapter—not an easy task since myotonic dystrophy is proving to be indeed a very complex condition. What I say here will definitely be an oversimplification and will in part become outdated quite soon—you should feel encouraged by this as it means that things are progressing quickly!

First, I should like to stress that much research depends directly on you, as patients and family members. This is not just through raising money for research, though this is indeed very important as laboratory work is extremely expensive. Your direct involvement is equally valuable, and indeed this has been essential over recent years in all the major advances that have occurred. This is a chance for me to say 'thank you' to all who have provided blood or tissue samples and family and other information, not just to my colleagues and myself, but to other groups involved in research worldwide. It is impossible to underestimate the value of this, now and in the future also. You can gain an impression of how much research is in progress by looking in my larger book *Myotonic dystrophy*, but I cannot possibly cover it all here. You should also feel encouraged by the extent to which research information is shared by different workers across the world; information obtained by one group is rapidly made available to others, and there is a close network of both laboratory scientists and clinical researchers who meet regularly to discuss their progress and new ideas.

Why, then, if this is so, is it such a long process unravelling the complexities of myotonic dystrophy and finding an effective treatment? I shall try to give you an idea here why this is the case; indeed myotonic dystrophy is one of the most complex disorders known to medicine, as you will already have appreciated from its variability and the range of body systems involved.

If we go back to the earlier years of research, this was mainly involving the clinical features of the disorder, the microscopic changes in muscle, heart, and other organs, and the inheritance pattern in families. All of this was important, but it left us a long way from understanding the primary cause of the condition. The real breakthrough came around 20 years ago, when new genetic techniques made it possible to map particular genes on a chromosome, to identify them and the specific change in a genetic disorder, and to work out from the genes themselves, what they normally do in the body and how this goes wrong in disease. I shall try to take you through this process step by step, and feel greatly privileged to have been part of this research effort throughout my professional life, and to have been able to make some contributions to it.

By the early 1980s we already knew that myotonic dystrophy was determined by one main gene, and that this was placed on chromosome 19, but this chromosome, though small, carries many hundreds of genes, so knowing this still left a long way to go. It took 10 years of very painstaking work before the myotonic dystrophy gene was finally pinned down and isolated in early 1992. At last research now could really take off.

At this point several remarkable and very important facts started to emerge. First, the genetic alteration (scientific term—mutation) was the same in almost all patients with myotonic dystrophy worldwide—quite unlike most inherited disorders where one often finds several hundred different mutations, differently distributed in different populations. This also had the great practical benefit that a single genetic blood test could be used for patients across the world—and it should be noted that the discoverers made it freely available for everyone to use.

Next, it became clear that the mutation was quite variable between patients, even within a family, something that immediately explained why the condition itself was so remarkably variable. Furthermore it was *unstable*, with a tendency to enlarge from generation to generation. This explained the questions relating to *anticipation*—the tendency to earlier onset in succeeding generations that had been noted for many years but which no one could explain.

I have already mentioned that the most severe and earliest onset patients are generally those with the largest change in the gene; here was another link between the genetic change and the clinical disorder and an explanation of why the condition is so variable.

All these findings resolved most of the puzzling genetic features of myotonic dystrophy, but a further important clue was the finding that the unstable part of the gene consisted of a series of repeated 'triplets', sets of three of the building blocks (chemicals) making up the DNA of the gene sequence. Whereas most people in the general population were found to have less than 30 of these triplets in a row, myotonic dystrophy patients showed over 50, usually several hundred, and in some severely affected children, several thousand. This 'repeat number' or 'repeat length' could be measured and now forms the basis for genetic tests in myotonic dystrophy. The actual components of the triplet are the building blocks C, T, and G, giving the triplet CTG. Figure 7.1 shows (very roughly) the difference between the normal situation and the enlargement in myotonic dystrophy.

Research workers now realized that myotonic dystrophy was not completely unique in showing a change of this kind. Several other genetic disorders proved around the same time to show an unstable 'triplet repeat' and all showed that same instability in a family as in myotonic dystrophy, though the actual diseases were very different in nature. They include Fragile-X chromosome, Huntington's disease, and others.

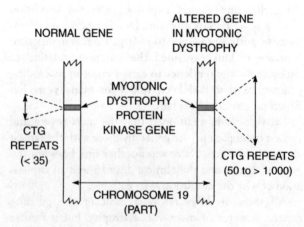

Figure 7.1 The genetic change in myotonic dystrophy

So within a year or two of the myotonic dystrophy gene being found, we had a clear explanation of its variability, the anticipation between generations and an accurate genetic test, all of real importance and of practical value to families. But how might this help us understand what the gene actually does and how the change in it produces myotonic dystrophy? This has proved much more complex and is still in the process of being resolved. Do not worry if you find the next few pages difficult to understand—everyone else has found this area confusing too, until very recently.

When researchers find a gene, the first thing they do is to determine its exact sequence, in terms of the four building blocks A, C, G, and T (adenine, cytosine, guanine, and thymidine) which make up the DNA molecule found in the nucleus of a cell. If one puts this sequence into a computer, then it may predict the type of protein the gene would be expected to make, which in turn can indicate its likely function in the body. When this was done for the myotonic dystrophy gene, it showed particular features suggesting a protein belonging to the 'protein kinase' family of proteins; hence it became known as myotonic dystrophy protein kinase or DMPK for short.

This seemed promising but the properties of DMPK proved not very specific and for a time confusing. Some workers found levels to be raised in myotonic dystrophy, others found them reduced. Likewise, it was not at first clear whether it was present just in muscle or throughout the body, or whether or not the nature of it was altered in myotonic dystrophy. Nor was it at all clear how DMPK could explain the features of the disorder. Sorting this out took several years and we are still not clear on all aspects. Table 7.1 shows how one can examine the abnormality at different levels.

What does seem definite now is that DMPK occurs mainly in muscle and heart, not elsewhere and that lack of it in an experimental animal does *not* cause muscle disease closely resembling myotonic dystrophy, though

Table 7.1 What goes wrong in myotonic dystrophy? The basic defect seen at different levels (see also Figure 7.1)

The gene (DNA)	Expansion of a 'triplet repeat' sequence on chromosome number 19. Nearby genes also possibly affected
The intermediate 'messenger' (RNA)	Trapped in the cell nucleus. Also binds to and affects other types of RNA
The proteins (the main components of body tissues)	Production of several different types affected (involving muscle, heart, and other organs)
The muscle (or other affected organ)	Key protein components faulty or deficient. Secondary damage from other factors

there are effects on heart conduction. So the conclusion has to be that while the myotonic dystrophy mutation is definitely in the DMPK gene, one probably cannot put all the clinical features of the disorder down to this protein alone.

While this work was in progress, others were looking to see what other explanations could be helpful. The first point to note is that the particular area of chromosome 19 is densely packed with genes and that at least two others lie immediately next to the DMPK gene. So perhaps the enlarged repeat sequence could be having an effect on their function and this might be involved in the features of myotonic dystrophy? Study of these genes has shown that one is especially involved in the lens of the eye, suggesting it might play a role in the cataract of myotonic dystrophy, but this remains to be proved. What did emerge was the idea that myotonic dystrophy might be the result of not just one, but of a group of adjacent genes not working properly—an attractive idea because of the multiple organs affected by the disorder.

A powerful research tool in all of this has been the study of 'transgenic' mice, where a normal or altered human gene has been introduced into the DNA of the mouse, allowing workers to study the effects in detail. This approach should also be of value in testing out new treatments for safety and effectiveness, as will be seen in the final chapter. By introducing an enlarged repeat sequence into such a mouse, we have now gained what seems to be the most promising model for how myotonic dystrophy occurs.

This mouse shows both myotonia and muscle disease, and the muscle changes resemble those seen in the muscle of myotonic dystrophy patients. Equally important, the effect of the repeat sequence seems not to be just on the DMPK or another single protein but on a series of important proteins. The way this happens appears to be as follows.

First the repeat in the DNA of the gene itself is turned into a comparable repeat in the intermediate molecule RNA, which is directly responsible for forming proteins. The building blocks are slightly altered so that the repeat is now CUG, not CTG, but it is otherwise similar. It seems now that this altered RNA is trapped inside the cell nucleus, affecting other types of RNA so that these are unable to produce proteins in the normal way. Some of the proteins involved are important in the heart, in handling insulin, and in other functions affected in myotonic dystrophy. Such a process would explain why so many different systems are affected in myotonic dystrophy—different proteins would indeed be involved, but the genes would not all have to be near each other.

This mechanism of producing disordered function has recently been given strong support by the identification of the gene for PROMM, also known as type 2 myotonic dystrophy (see p. 14). The gene is on a different chromosome (3) and shows no resemblance to the DMPK gene or others near it, but it does contain a very large repeat (CCTG) in patients, suggesting that it is the actual mutation that is important rather than the gene it is in. The similarities (and differences) probably result from which particular proteins are affected by the trapped RNA in the nucleus.

At present scientists are still debating which of these mechanisms is most important in causing myotonic dystrophy—it is quite possible that a combination of them will be involved —and it is too early to be dogmatic. What is important is that research is now progressing very rapidly, and is bringing us closer to the point of giving us real targets for testing out approaches to treatment.

If you think back 10 years and realize that at that point we knew almost nothing of the processes underlying myotonic dystrophy, then I think you will agree that we have come a long way. With everyone's support and encouragement this can continue further until it reaches the point of giving real help to patients.

8
Support and information

If you have read this book up to this point, you should have learnt a lot about myotonic dystrophy, its associated problems, its genetic aspects, and even something about its causes. But you will not so far have found much that tells you what can be done about helping with the different problems myotonic dystrophy causes, nor about overall management and treatment. These last three chapters try to cover this area, the most important to you as a patient. I have written this chapter on support and information as separate to the others, because it is so often neglected or omitted in medically orientated works. Support can come from a range of sources (Table 8.1) and I shall say something about each of them.

Support from family and friends

This is the most natural form of support that people with myotonic dystrophy can receive—indeed so natural that it is all too often forgotten or taken for granted. If all the support given by family on a day-by-day basis over many years were to be suddenly removed, society would rapidly collapse. Unfortunately, not all people have this support, or it may be lost due to death of a parent or partner, or because of divorce. Some people find it very difficult to

Table 8.1 Myotonic dystrophy—sources of support

Family and friends
Support groups
Wider muscular dystrophy associations
Disability groups
Social support agencies

accept help and support, especially from wider family or friends. But overall the family remains the main source of support for most patients.

This makes it all the more important to recognize that carers and family members need support themselves. They may feel threatened by being at risk of the disorder themselves, by loss of income in the family, or by being tied to a severely affected patient without the chance of relief. It is natural for people to want to achieve their own aims in life without everything revolving around the disorder. It is often difficult to resolve such a situation, but at least it helps for it to be recognized. I hope also that this book will be of some help to family and carers in making clear the problems of myotonic dystrophy.

Friends may find it especially difficult to continue to be close to someone who may perhaps not be able to join in shared activities. They may be uncertain whether or when to mention myotonic dystrophy, or be worried that they will cause upset. Again, close friends will generally benefit from knowing more about the disorder.

Support groups

I am in no doubt that the information and development of support groups has been of the greatest importance for many disorders, especially those that are less frequent and less well recognized. Myotonic dystrophy is an excellent example of this, and I have no hesitation in saying that most patients and their families will gain just as much benefit from joining such a group as from anything doctors have to offer. My own experience has come from the activities of the UK group, but similar support groups are increasingly developing in other countries. What are the special things that support groups have to offer?

First is the realization that one is no longer alone, and that myotonic dystrophy is a problem that affects many other people and families. This will come not only as a relief, but often as a surprise, since most families will not have come across another affected family in their immediate neighbourhood or town. Even if you do nothing further, merely knowing that you are part of a wider group of people with the same condition can be a great help.

The next benefit is access to accurate and relevant information. The support group is often the first source of this, or at least the first source of information clearly relevant to you. This still applies even in the age of the Internet (see below), from which people may receive information which they may find confusing or difficult to interpret.

A third valuable area of help that support groups can supply is practical suggestions for dealing with problems of the disorder like mobility, other daily activities, or more specific problems. Since some of these problems may not be helped greatly by medical measures, the experience of individual patients and families in dealing with them can be especially helpful. This help often comes as contributions or notes in newsletters or at meetings.

Personal contact in the form of larger or more local meetings is an important role of support groups. A large annual meeting often becomes an enjoyable social event in the calendar, and can result also in close individual friendship. Naturally, some people are more social in temperament than others; it can at first be disturbing to meet a group of other people who have 'your' condition, especially if they have it more severely, but on the whole many people gain real value from these meetings.

A most important function of support groups is to provide an information network on what medical and other facilities are available in an area, and to promote their improvement. While larger associations are usually required if change is to come on a national basis, support groups are best placed to tap the personal experience of patients and families as to which doctors and clinics in a particular area are most knowledgeable and helpful— and which are best avoided. It is often possible for one or two active families to create real interest among doctors and other professionals that was lacking before because of unawareness or lack of information about myotonic dystrophy. It is always best to take a gradual and tactful approach when doing this, and if one has the backing and information from a support group, this makes the task easier.

The essential characteristic of support groups is that they are run 'by' as well as 'for' patients and their families. They may have professionals as advisers or helping in specific ways, but it is important that they do not dominate the group or interfere in its running. In the same way, support groups will often have many members keen to promote and take part in research, but it is essential that research workers do not take unfair advantage of this.

Since support groups generally have personal links and relatively small size as helpful features, it follows that there are some functions that are better undertaken by larger organizations with more infrastructure and administrative support. This is where the broader associations involved with muscular dystrophies in general have a particularly important role.

Broader muscular dystrophy associations

The support available to myotonic dystrophy patients and family members from these complements the functions of the support groups. They are generally organized on a national scale and examples are the Muscular Dystrophy Association of America, the Association contre les Myopathies (AFM; France), and the Muscular Dystrophy Campaign (UK). Web and postal addresses are given in Appendix 1. As a result of their larger income and professional fund-raising activities, these bodies are better placed than support groups to fund research, especially expensive laboratory research. Also they will usually have an independent scientific committee to ensure that applications for grants are assessed thoroughly.

Production of literature is also possible on a larger scale than support groups can usually manage. Thus, in the UK helpful booklets on myotonic dystrophy are available as well as a comprehensive book on disability aids. Funding of professional family care workers in different regions has proved of great value as a link between patients and medical facilities.

The disadvantage of these larger associations is that they need to cover a wide range of very different muscle conditions, so it is difficult to focus specifically on any one; this is why the support groups and the larger bodies each have valuable and distinct roles.

Other helpful bodies

At an international level it is important to have close links between countries, especially in helping smaller countries or those with less well-developed facilities. The European Alliance of Muscular Dystrophy Associations (EAMDA), acting as a federation, along with the European Neuromuscular Centre (ENMC), has been valuable in organizing small expert group meetings for different muscular dystrophies, including myotonic dystrophy and PROMM.

When it comes to political lobbying, a combined approach is also more effective than separate approaches by numerous small societies. In the UK, the Genetic Interest

Group (GIG), which represents over 100 separate disease associations, has been extremely effective in promoting services for genetic disorders, while a range of disability groups has fought hard on issues which are shared by different disorders, such as mobility, access, and education.

The Internet and information

With many (probably most in some countries) families having Internet access, this has become a powerful tool in helping myotonic dystrophy patients. At a practical level it allows shopping and purchasing of a range of items to be easily done for those whose mobility is restricted. Equally, it is now becoming the main provider of information on medical aspects of many conditions, including myotonic dystrophy.

Because the amount of information is growing so rapidly, I have listed only a very few sources here (see Appendix 1) and have not tried to be comprehensive. A recent search showed over 4000 different entries related to myotonic dystrophy, some quite extensive.

This huge amount of information now means that very few people are completely without information, but the problem now arises of how to select from it and how to know what is accurate, appropriate, and relevant to yourself. A colleague has described the situation as like 'trying to drink from a fire hydrant'—you can get knocked over by the sheer volume and pressure of information.

In using the material you have to remember that it is not filtered, checked, or censored—so it may or may not be accurate. You should be very cautious in making any information about yourself available—it will be open to the whole world. Likewise, while informal conversation groups can be very valuable for people who have mobility problems, who live in remote areas, or who are shy of face-to-face contact in support groups, you should be cautious in how you use them.

In conclusion, there is now a lot of support and information available for you and your family. Much of the information is clear and valuable, and there are numerous helpful and well-informed people who can help you. You should no longer feel alone, and by using the support wisely you will both be able to benefit from it—and also to help others in a similar situation.

9
Management and treatment now

Many people with myotonic dystrophy, who have just been diagnosed and have asked what treatment can be given, have been discouraged to be told 'nothing'. While this remains true at present as regards a cure or medical treatment that will radically affect the course of the condition, it is most definitely not true in terms of measures that can be helpful, even life-saving, at many points in the course of the disorder. Specific symptoms can also be treated as they arise. The final chapter of this book looks at the prospects for definitive or curative treatment, but in this chapter I deal with what can be done here and now, which all patients with myotonic dystrophy should have access to.

At many points in this book I have emphasized the variability of myotonic dystrophy; this means that different patients will need different approaches according to how severe particular problems are, and also depending on their age. Since age does make a considerable difference, I have considered management of adults and children separately, though there is considerable overlap. I have summarized much of the information in tables and cross-referred to the earlier chapters covering the different problems. You may find it useful to photocopy some of the tables to take with you if you are meeting doctors or professionals to discuss management.

Muscle symptoms

See Table 9.1. At present muscle stiffness due to myotonia is the only muscle symptom that might require and respond to specific drug treatment, and this is only needed by a minority of people. Remember that the myotonia will be with you for many years, and that even though side-effects are infrequent, it can occur over a long period of time. The most frequently used drug now is mexilitene, but some patients prefer to continue with older drugs such as phenytoin, quinine, or procainamide. The doses are best determined by your doctor. Most of these drugs can have some depressant effect on heart conduction (though they are also used outside muscle disease for treating heart problems), so if you have heart disease, they are best avoided or used only under close supervision. Phenytoin in excess may cause unsteadiness; it also may cause damage to the baby during pregnancy, so if you are pregnant or (just as important) likely to become pregnant, it is best to avoid all medication for myotonia.

Muscle weakness is at present not helped by any drug, though agents under trial or emerging in the future will hopefully alter this situation. It is wise to give a warning

Table 9.1 Treatment of muscle symptoms in myotonic dystrophy

Problem	Treatment/management
Muscle stiffness (myotonia)	Drugs only if symptoms troublesome (see text)
Leg and foot weakness	Plastic ankle splints; foot spring
Neck weakness	Fitted soft collar; head support in cars, chairs
Drooping eyelids	Elevating spectacles (rarely surgery)
General weakness	Wheelchair (especially powered, for outdoor use)

here that it is best not to use medicines that have been reported as helping other muscle conditions in the hope that they could help you too. It is unlikely that they will, and quite possible that they might cause harm. This applies to steroids of various types, to high doses of different vitamins and minerals, and to herbal and other traditional remedies. Remember that 'natural' medicines may be as toxic as artificial ones—for example foxglove and deadly nightshade!

Diet has already been mentioned in Chapter 3 in terms of excess weight gain; there is no evidence that dietary factors can specifically improve muscle strength, and while a generally nourishing diet is sensible, there is little point in spending extra money on special diets in the hope that they will improve your muscles.

Exercise is often enquired about and again has been mentioned earlier. It is certainly important in keeping generally healthy and mobile, but strenuous activities such as long distance running or weight lifting are likely to do more harm than good (though I have to say that there is little objective evidence on this). Swimming is found helpful by many since the water takes much of one's weight. Do not attempt to lose weight by increasing exercise as an alternative to reducing your calorie intake—this is rarely successful.

If you cannot make your muscles stronger you can at least, by careful planning, take some of the strain off them. Here we come back to commonsense measures—but it is surprising how frequently they are not used. In terms of general mobility the needs of myotonic dystrophy patients are to some extent similar to those of other patients with muscle problems and are best assessed by an expert in this area; this will usually be an occupational therapist, often working closely with a physiotherapist. Often now, such experts are based in centres where needs can be fully assessed more easily than in a clinic, and where a full range of appliances and disability aids can be tried out. It is important for all involved to know that myotonic dystrophy usually causes mobility problems more through weakness of the lower legs and feet than through involvement of the large weight-bearing muscles. This may alter the approach needed.

Driving is of particular importance if your muscle weakness is preventing you from walking distances and public transport is poor. You should think carefully whether your car needs adapting; before changing it, try to get expert advice on the type that is most suited. Also remember that weakness of the neck muscles makes it especially important to have a good supporting headrest; this applies equally to passengers as to the driver.

Weakness of particular muscles can also be helped; thus foot drop, a common problem due to weakness at the ankles, can be corrected by wearing light moulded plastic splints that fit inside the shoes and which cannot be seen. A soft neck collar, as used by people with other neck problems, can be useful, especially if neck pain or headache are associated with the neck weakness. Drooping eyelids can be supported by special spectacles.

Aids and appliances in the home

Trying to help your muscle weakness should not stop with adaptations that involve your body; you should examine your surroundings, too, to see how they might be altered to help you. This mainly means your home, but your workplace is also important. Adaptations to avoid injury are clearly vital and have been mentioned already, but such changes will also avoid strain and effort and will stop you becoming easily tired.

Any major changes of this type need planning with expert advice—again the skill of an occupational therapist or a disability living centre will be helpful. They also need thought and planning well in advance—do not put things off until a crisis occurs.

Finally, if your weakness is severe and your mobility increasingly restricted, have you considered use of a wheelchair, particularly for use outdoors or on unfamiliar terrain? I have found that initially many people are reluctant even to think about the possibility, even though they may have had to stop doing many of the activities they most enjoy; a wheelchair, especially a powered one, could allow them to continue these and remain relatively independent. I use the analogy to such reluctant people of our ancestors a few generations ago who were reluctant to use modern inventions such as the car or the train. How many people would now think of walking from one town to another? Usually, once people see for themselves how they can benefit, it is easier to accept the use of a wheelchair, or any other mobility aid. For most myotonic dystrophy patients it will not be essential, but it should not be dismissed.

Medical problems

I have already stressed that the various medical problems which can be associated with myotonic dystrophy can for some people be as or even more troublesome than muscle weakness, and that, if not recognized and treated, they can be dangerous, even for those without severe muscle symptoms. It is vital that these general aspects are checked on a regular basis and not neglected by neurologists and other specialists in muscle disease.

Table 9.2 summarizes the most important medical problems that can need management and treatment; they are dealt with more fully in Chapter 4, so only a few comments about the types of treatment are given here.

Heart problems

The treatment required will depend on the type of rhythm disturbance and is best determined by a heart specialist. If drugs do not restore or maintain regular

Table 9.2 Management and treatment. Medical Problems

Heart	Regular ECGs; more detailed investigation if needed. Specific drugs to correct heart rhythm; heart pacemaker if indicated.
Chest	Avoid food or liquid entering lungs. Prompt antibiotics for infections. Assisted ventilation at night if needed.
Bowel problems	'Antispasmodic' drugs for abdominal pain and 'irritable bowel' symptoms
Daytime sleepiness	Exclude poor breathing function. Specific agents under trial
Diabetes	Diet modifications; insulin not often needed.
Cataract	Good results from surgical removal.

rhythm, electrical treatment may be needed for this, while for slow conduction ('heart block') an artificial pacemaker may be needed. There is considerable debate as to whether this last is best inserted before symptoms occur or whether to wait. Incidentally if these procedures sound alarming, you should remember that they are often used in very elderly or frail patients, have good results, and in any case will only be needed in a minority of people with myotonic dystrophy.

Lung problems

If these are due to food 'going the wrong way', then the solution is to recognize and stop this. Adjusting the diet, in conjunction with a speech and swallowing therapist, can help, as can preventing food running back from the stomach by not sleeping flat and avoiding a large, late evening meal.

If it is the weakness of breathing muscles at night that is the cause, then these can be helped by wearing a device that stimulates night breathing, though this is not often required. It is important for any bronchitis or throat infection to be treated at once with antibiotics to avoid the infection 'going to the chest', something that is more likely to happen if the cough is weak. Again, a physiotherapist may be able to instruct you in breathing exercises that keep the chest clear.

Bowel problems and abdominal pain

These can be helped by various drugs that relax the muscle of the bowel wall, as in the common condition 'irritable bowel'. A high-fibre diet may be helpful and if constipation is being treated, it is important to avoid liquid paraffin (less used now anyway) since it can be especially damaging if it enters the lungs.

Daytime sleepiness

This is a troublesome symptom for which trials are currently in progress using several drugs, so it is worth enquiring as to the progress of these.

Diabetes

Diabetes occurs in only a small proportion of myotonic dystrophy patients and is often of the type not requiring insulin. If it is present, though, good control is even more important than for other diabetics; you do not want to add unnecessarily to your other health problems.

Cataracts

Finally, cataracts are removable surgically with excellent results, even in those who are in poor health or who are elderly.

Of course, there are numerous rare complications of myotonic dystrophy that I have not mentioned here; in general their treatment is no different from when the problem occurs without myotonic dystrophy. However, it is always important for whoever is treating the particular problem to know that you have myotonic dystrophy, otherwise they may risk making other aspects of your disorder worse.

Surgery and anaesthesia

All of us need this at some points in our life, whether as the result of illness or accident. If you have myotonic dystrophy, then there is no reason why you, too, should not benefit from them—but they must be used with the greatest caution, and in the knowledge that you have myotonic dystrophy. There are several points that you and your doctors should consider.

1. Do you really need surgery? You should think carefully whether it is going to make a big difference to your life, whether there are non-surgical alternatives, and whether the surgical diagnosis is really right. Could the symptoms (for example, abdominal pain) be related to your myotonic dystrophy and best dealt with medically? If you really do need surgery, then the next question should be as below.

2. Where should the surgery be done? The simple answer is only in a hospital that has proper back-up facilities, including intensive care if something were to go badly wrong. This applies especially to relatively simpler procedures, which may be carried out in private or other settings without such back up—this may be all right if you are a healthy person but *not* if you have myotonic dystrophy. In the UK there is no substitute for a proper National Health Service hospital with junior staff on call at night—even if you do already have private insurance.

3. Surgeon and anaesthetist must know about your condition *in advance*. There is no point in telling

them on your way to the operating theatre! Likewise, they must realize the potential hazards so they can plan the necessary facilities and procedures.

4. What needs to be done before, during, and after the operation? This will vary according to the type of operation and anaesthesia, so it is unwise to lay down fixed rules. I have given in Appendix 2 the procedures worked out by anaesthetic and other colleagues in our centre; although technical, you should be able to copy it and give it to those involved.

5. Surgery in emergencies. If you have a car accident or other emergency there may be no time for any of the planning outlined above, but if you carry a warning card or bracelet stating clearly that you have myotonic dystrophy, this will alert staff to the problem. The UK Myotonic Dystrophy Support Group now have a wallet size plastic card and a folding sheet that gives a basic set of information (see Appendix 3).

Childbirth

Problems of pregnancy and delivery have been mentioned in Chapter 6, but if you have myotonic dystrophy and are pregnant, it is important to recognize that caesarean section or anaesthesia are common outcomes, so it is essential for you, as well as for your baby, that you are delivered in a hospital with full facilities.

Management overall

You will have recognized from this chapter that it will be easier and more effective if the various aspects of managing and treating your myotonic dystrophy are coordinated, rather than being dealt with piecemeal by a series of different specialists. Naturally, it will often require a specialist in the field to deal with such problems as cataract or heart complications, but these specialists will not really be able to manage or coordinate your condition as a whole.

In the UK, where everyone is registered with a family doctor, this is still the best person to act as coordinator, even though most family doctors are greatly under pressure. To get the best help from your family doctor, it is better not to wait until you are ill but to arrange to see them to introduce yourself and your disorder. Take along relevant literature so it can be put in your file (but only one or two pages!) and discuss whether a regular appointment and necessary tests (electrocardiogram, ECG) are best arranged with the practice or with a hospital clinic. Remember that most practices have nurses attached to them who may prove the best link and who may be more used to arranging such matters as occupational therapy assessments and social benefits. If the practice staff are familiar with both you yourself and the problems of your disorder, then you are much more likely to get informed help when you are ill. Most doctors will also be genuinely interested in your condition, which they will not have met often before. Remember also that it is the family doctor who will have most information about the different specialists in your locality, and will best know who to recommend.

At the level of hospital care, you may be able to have access to a specialist muscle clinic; if it handles considerable numbers of myotonic dystrophy patients, then it will certainly be a helpful contact point and source of expert help. Unfortunately there are only few such clinics, so they cannot possibly see all myotonic dystrophy patients on a regular basis, but they are the best place for having your muscle condition regularly assessed and for asking about new developments.

Ideally the best combination is to have an interested family doctor with associated staff and occasional visits (perhaps once a year) to a specialist muscle clinic, with specific problems being handled by whichever specialty is appropriate. Add to this, contact with an active support group at local and national level and you should have a satisfactory framework for helping you with most of the problems that may arise from your disorder. Unfortunately, only a few people actually get this ideal service, but it is something to aim and campaign for; if you have a system that works well in some areas, it is always easier to convince those planning health services that their area should not be deficient.

To conclude, there is a lot that can be done in the management and treatment of specific aspects of myotonic dystrophy which can greatly help you, as an affected person, even in the absence of a cure. Some of the points mentioned require medical help, both from specialists in particular fields and for overall coordination. But there is a large amount that you yourself can do, or at least initiate, if you are well informed about your condition; you can take a sensible attitude in avoiding likely pitfalls and you can be prepared to be persistent, but patient and cooperative with the various medical and other professional staff whose help you will need, and who may well know less about myotonic dystrophy than you do. The suggestions outlined in this chapter should help to keep you in as good condition as possible, so that when an effective treatment for myotonic dystrophy is discovered, you will be able to take best advantage of it.

10 The future—towards effective prevention and cure for myotonic dystrophy

At the time of writing this there is no proven medical treatment that influences the rate at which myotonic dystrophy deteriorates overall, or which can prevent its onset in those carrying the genetic change.

This must seem a discouraging statement with which to start the final chapter of this book, but it is best to be honest at the outset, before looking at why and how this situation is likely to change. I have already shown you how many things can be done that can help in particular areas in the absence of specific treatment, but all these are essentially interim measures until something effective is found that can alter the course of the condition. I am more optimistic now than at any time over the past 30 years that I have been involved with myotonic dystrophy, so in this chapter, I should like to indicate why, and where advances seem most likely to be of practical help.

Understanding and research

Chapter 7 outlined where we stand at present; it is easy to forget that until less than 10 years ago we had absolutely no idea as to the nature of the genetic change underlying myotonic dystrophy, while it is only during the past 2–3 years that we are starting to be able to connect up this change with how the damage to muscle and other systems actually occurs.

This would not have happened without research, much of it based in laboratories, but also involving clinical research on people like you and your family. Much of this has at times seemed frustrating, even discouraging, but it has been the goal of understanding how things work—and go wrong—with the hope of leading ultimately to effective treatment, that has kept scientists and clinical workers going. It is probably true to say that 1992 was a watershed in this process; once the gene and its mutation were discovered, it was clear that it must be only a matter of time, hard work, and persistence that would allow the details of what goes wrong in myotonic dystrophy to be understood, and that this could then be the starting point for work on treatment.

Could a cure for myotonic dystrophy appear without this long process of increasing understanding through research? In my view this is very unlikely, though not absolutely impossible. Most claims for new medical treatments not based on clear facts or evidence prove to be illusions. There have been numerous such poorly founded claims for other muscular dystrophies, but none have stood up to rigorous testing, and there have been many disappointed patients and families as a result. There is likely to be no short cut, however frustrating delay may seem.

It is important though to recognize that it is not just research on myotonic dystrophy itself that is going to prove helpful. Work on other types of muscle disease can give key insights on what is happening in myotonic dystrophy, while basic 'blue skies' research on mechanisms of normal processes can also be of the greatest importance—even though those doing the work may have never heard of myotonic dystrophy! This is why it is important that all those involved in research keep in close contact and meet to exchange ideas—you never know where the next important advance might come from.

Which advances in research are most likely to result in treatment?

From this point I am going to have to speculate, so I may very well be proved wrong. But there is no harm in sharing my thoughts, providing you recognize that they are only thoughts, and that I am mainly a clinical worker, not a laboratory scientist.

Therapy at the gene level

Let us start with the genetic change or 'mutation' and ask if we are likely to be able to correct this? We have seen that virtually all myotonic dystrophy patients have the same genetic change; enlargement of a 'triplet repeat' sequence in a particular part of a specific gene. Very broadly the larger the expansion of this the worse will be the disorder, so could we alter this in some way?

In fact this can happen occasionally in nature, since individuals have been documented who have clearly inherited the 'abnormal' copy of the gene from their affected parent, yet are quite healthy. This is because the enlarged repeat sequence has decreased again into the normal range. Could one somehow make this happen in a patient? With all the publicity given to gene therapy it might seem possible to replace the altered gene with a normal copy and so prevent the condition from developing.

Unfortunately this is not in my view a likely possibility, for several reasons. First, unless the change were made in a very early embryo there would be no way of correcting the change throughout the body, while simply adding a normal copy—say to muscle—later in life would not be likely to help since all the evidence suggests that it is not lack of a normal gene that causes the problem. After all, every myotonic dystrophy patient already has one normal copy as well as an altered one, yet this does not prevent the condition from developing. So I doubt if any form of 'gene therapy' is going to help significantly.

Changing the RNA

This next approach is perhaps the most exciting and could provide an entirely novel approach to treatment. For those of you who have forgotten (since Chapter 7) what RNA is, it is the intermediate chemical between the gene itself (made of DNA) and the proteins, which actually control body functions. We saw in Chapter 7 that one of the results of the expanded repeat sequence in myotonic dystrophy seems to be to affect the production of RNA molecules in the cell nucleus by binding to them and that this can involve a range of different types of RNA that produce key proteins necessary for the function of muscle, heart, and other systems. If one could devise ways of stopping this process, then the different types of RNA could get out of the nucleus and produce the different proteins normally.

This approach is so new that it would be unwise to expect it to provide any rapid advances in treatment, but now that it is recognized it is an area that can be worked on—a good example of how vital it is to understand the processes involved. Already people are studying animal models, where an expanded repeat sequence has been introduced, so that the process of RNA trapping and how it can be modified can be investigated. We will have to await the results of these studies before patients are studied.

Treatment at the protein level

I have already indicated that myotonic dystrophy— unlike some genetic conditions—is not simply the result of a single protein being deficient, which might be replaced in some way. However, now that it is becoming clearer that several different proteins are likely to be involved, probably because involvement of the RNA for each of them stops them being made adequately, it should become possible to work out which particular protein is involved in any particular aspect of the disorder—muscle, heart, eye, and so on—and focus on how that particular protein can be made to work better. It could turn out that this will be more feasible than trying to modify the RNA, especially as we already know quite a lot about some of the proteins that seem to be involved. It would not surprise me if some trials of therapy based on this approach become feasible during the next 5 years or so.

Research on animals

Everyone would wish to avoid this if it were possible, but it needs to be faced that for many lines of research, including some of the most important, use of animals is essential. This is especially the case for 'transgenic' animal models, where it is now possible to introduce the genetic change for a human disorder, such as myotonic dystrophy, into an animal (usually a mouse) and study the effects. This could not ethically or for safety reasons be done on human volunteers, and some of the most promising recent advances in our understanding of myotonic dystrophy have come from this approach. When the next stage is reached of assessing new agents for treatment, such animal models will be of equal importance in seeing whether the agent works and whether there are harmful effects or not.

At the same time it should be recognized that genetic research has allowed much animal experimentation to be avoided. Thus, because our genetic makeup is so similar to that of all living organisms, much basic research relevant to myotonic dystrophy has been able to be done on simple organisms such as yeasts or bacteria rather than on mammals. Equally, cell culture techniques allow human cells to be studied outside the body. But it would be wrong to conclude that animal experiments can now be avoided if we are to understand and find effective treatments for myotonic dystrophy; they cannot, and this needs to be recognized by all who wish for improved treatment and understanding of complex genetic disorders.

Trials of new treatments

This brings us to the next stage that needs to be thought about; once we have some reasonable evidence about the various steps that go wrong in myotonic dystrophy and can identify agents that seem to show effects in animal models and basic cell processes, how can we start to try these out on patients with myotonic dystrophy?

This is where it is very important that you realize that there are well-recognized procedures, similar for all new treatments in medicine, that need to be gone through before a new treatment can be accepted as effective. These are time consuming, expensive, and often disappointing in the end, but the alternative of simply trying something new out in a haphazard way has proved far more unsatisfactory over the years, with initial enthusiasm giving way to uncertainty and confusion, and even with danger to patients.

I have summarized some of the main points of such trials in Table 10.1. You may well be unaware that such a complex process is needed, but it will help you understand why something new cannot simply be made available right away. The first point to be made is that there has to be reasonable evidence before even starting a full evaluation. It is irresponsible to demand a trial just because of a 'hunch' or even because of a single patient's response; a proper trial will cost many thousands of pounds and assessing something with no real evidence behind it may mean that funds are diverted from something more soundly based.

Table 10.1 Clinical trials for new treatments—some important steps

Evidence from basic research—is it adequate?
Safety—is this known from animals or humans?
Effects aimed for—can they be measured?
Numbers of patients needed—single centre or many?
'Control' group for comparison
Analysing results—how do we know there is significant benefit?

Safety is obviously vital—the old adage for doctors 'first do no harm' is as important today as in the past. Of course, it may be that what is being tried out is a drug already used for other medical conditions and known to be safe, but if it is completely new then rigorous checks, first on animals, then on patients will be needed.

Once the stage of a proper trial is reached, then one has to think carefully of what the aims are and how one measures any effects. If the aim is to improve muscle weakness, then it is not much use just assessing myotonia. Also, for a slowly changing disorder like myotonic dystrophy, it is essential to have a long time period if one is to see any real change, especially if the likely effect is to stop weakness from getting worse rather than improving it. This also influences the numbers involved; unless the effects are dramatic (not likely) many more patients are often needed than you might think; help from statisticians is essential and increasingly multi-centre trials are needed to get sufficient numbers. The same statistical help is needed to know when a clear result is reached—which is hopefully of benefit but it could be important to know when to stop the trial if it is making people worse.

Almost all trials need to have some comparison or 'control' group that is not receiving the treatment. This is because just being in a trial may make patients feel better, or it may give access to improved general management. The only way around this is for one group in the trial to be receiving a dummy or 'placebo' treatment, and for neither patient nor doctor to know until the code is broken.

What I have outlined here about trials has assumed that it is the study of the general overall effect on the condition, especially the progress of muscle weakness, that is being aimed at. But trials are equally valuable for more limited aims related to specific symptoms, and some are in progress now. Symptoms such as daytime sleepiness or abdominal symptoms are examples where control of these symptoms would be of real help, even if the treatment did not affect the disorder overall. A trials framework can and should be used for studying these symptoms as well as for assessing more curative treatment.

Preparing for trials now

You can see from what I have outlined above, that even when research starts to produce promising agents to try out, whether drugs or other approaches, the process of assessing them is complex and time consuming. Trials cannot simply be set up overnight. It is therefore very important that the foundations are put in place now. This essentially means having research orientated clinics with the additional staff and time that can allow detailed assessments over a period of years and which are linked with other clinics, often internationally, so that everyone is following a similar pattern. Then, when something promising does become available, there is a proper foundation on which it can be based.

Sadly it has proved very difficult, at least in the UK, to persuade any of the funding organizations involved to show interest or support at the stage before there is a specific substance available to be tried. Although informal networks have been set up, these can only function well if there is a series of clinics properly funded and coordinated for this, over and above the level needed to provide existing services. It is only strong pressure from support groups working internationally and alongside those involved with other types of muscular dystrophy that is likely to make things happen. In the USA, things are rather more advanced.

On the other hand, one of the most encouraging aspects of work in the field of myotonic dystrophy is the close cooperation and comradeship of all those working on the disorder. This has shown itself during the long period of work in identifying the genetic basis, and is again equally evident in preparing for trials. The number and range of interests of scientists working on myotonic dystrophy has increased hugely from the small band that existed before the gene defect was known, and the links between laboratory and clinical scientists are probably closer than ever before. Since the contacts and links are international, any advance made in one part of the world will have immediate impact in other countries, as was shown in practical fashion by the way in which use of the genetic change for gene testing was made immediately available across the world without restrictions or charges. Now that the focus of all involved is on finding effective treatment, you can expect that, if given the financial support and general encouragement from the different organizations involved, the scientists and clinicians working on myotonic dystrophy will continue to make steady progress towards finding agents that will have a real effect on the underlying course of the disorder.

11
Conclusion

I have reached the end of this book and am conscious that there is a lot more that I could have included and that much of what I have said may not be altogether clearly written. I also recognize that people will be looking for what neither I nor anyone else can give at present—a promise of effective treatment in the immediate future.

Despite this, I hope that, for some of you at least, this short book will have given you a clearer picture of your own disorder and also will have provided some practical suggestions for how you can best help yourself—and your doctors. I have tried to combine both a realistic and an optimistic approach, being firmly convinced that while there are very real hopes from future advances—greater in my view than at any time before—there are also numerous helpful steps that can be taken now. Most of the practical aspects I have outlined will apply wherever in the world you live; and I greatly hope that the book will also help to ensure that, for those living where health care is less well provided, standards of care for myotonic dystrophy patients and families can progressively be brought up to the standard of what is available to those in more fortunate countries.

The future lies not just in the hands of research scientists, clinicians, and other professionals, but in your own hands as patients, support groups, and international bodies; working closely together will certainly increase the speed of progress. I expect and greatly hope that this progress will make much of what I have written here rapidly outdated.

Finally, writing this gives me the opportunity of saying that being able to work with myotonic dystrophy patients and families for a period of over 30 years has been both a pleasure and a privilege. I have often been conscious of how little I have been able to help on particular occasions, but this is a chance to record my thanks to you all in the form of this book.

Appendix 1

Support groups and organizations

Association Française contre les Myopathies (AFM)
1, Rue de l'Internationale, BP59, 91002 Evry,
France
Especially valuable for people living in France or in other French-speaking countries.

European Alliance of Muscular Dystrophy Associations (EAMDA)
E-mail: mail@eamda.sonnet.co.uk

European Neuromuscular Centre (ENMC)
Sponsor of a valuable series of small workshops on neuromuscular disorders, including myotonic dystrophy.

Muscular Dystrophy Association of America (MDA)
3300 East Sunrise Drive, Tucson, Arizona, AZ 85718–3208,
USA
www.mdausa.org
www.mdausa.org/disease/dm.html (specific myotonic dystrophy page)

Muscular Dystrophy Campaign (UK)
7–11 Prescott Place, London, SW4 6BS,
UK
www.muscular-dystrophy.org
E-mail: info@muscular-dystrophy.org

Myotonic Dystrophy Support Group (UK)
www.mdsguk.org
E-mail: Mdsg@tesco.net
A specific support group for myotonic dystrophy patients and families, able to provide much practical information and help.

Appendix 2

Anaesthetic considerations in myotonic dystrophy

99th ENMC Workshop 10/11/01

Mark T. Rogers and Paul Clyburn
(University Hospital of Wales, Cardiff)

Anaesthesia can pose a serious risk to the myotonic patient. Most complications can be anticipated and avoided by careful pre-operative assessment, avoidance of certain drugs, and good post-operative management.

Anaesthetic considerations

i.   myotonia
ii.   temporomandibular subluxation
iii. cardiac dysrhythmias, cardiac failure (cardio-myopathy)
iv.   hypotension
v.   respiratory depression
vi.   somnolence—central and obstructive sleep apnoea
vii. swallowing difficulties
viii. cardiac sphincter dysfunction
ix.   diabetes mellitus

Which subsets of patients are most at risk?

- symptomatic but undiagnosed (therefore unexpected)
- moderate and severely affected
- the pregnant patient

Consider alternative methods to reduce risk

- local anaesthesia
- regional anaesthesia
  - spinal
  - epidural
  - nerve block
  - intravenous regional anaesthesia
- laparoscopy

Anaesthetic principles: pre-operative

- good pre-op assessment and workup
- avoid sedative premed

Anaesthetic principles: intra-operative

- minimal inhalational anaesthetic to avoid post-op shivering
- warming pad, warm fluids
- avoid K^+-containing fluids
- avoid depolarizing NMJ blockers
- use short acting non-depolarizing NMJ blockers (e.g. atracurium or vecuronium)
- (so avoid need for neostigmine and occasional paradoxical

depolarizing blockade—one
case report)

- protect airway and minimize
risks of aspiration, especially
in pregnant patients

Anaesthetic principles: analgesia and post-op

- analgesia
- avoid or minimal use of
opiates (patient self-
administration has been tried
with reported success) (not
forgetting potential effect on
congenitally affected
neonate)
- intra-operative local
anaesthesia
- epidural or regional
anaesthesia (including
post-op)
- TNS
- Automatic post-op initial
HDU/automatic chest
physiotherapy

Anticipate potential complications

- aspiration (ranitidine, cricoid
pressure during intubation)
- post-partum haemorrhage

A suggested anaesthetic protocol

Based on Bennun *et al.* (2000)
Br. J. Anaesth. **85**, 407–9.

Pre-op
- FBC
- biochem inx
- ECHO
- ECG
- lung function tests

- no pre-anaesthetic
medication
- anaesthetic room supine VC
and tidal volume
- intubate to protect airway

Intra-op monitoring
i.   ECG
ii. non-invasive arterial
pressure
iii. pulse oximetry
iv. capnograph
v.   nerve stimulator
vi. rectal temperature

Induction
i.   Fenatanyl 0.05 mg
ii. Propofol 2.5 mg/kg
iii. Atracurium 0.5 mg/kg

Maintenance
i. N_2O 70%
ii. propofol 6 mg/kg per h
iii. bolus fentanyl 2?g/kg
iv. incremental atracurium
0.2 mg/kg
v.   > 20% decrease in BP—
5 mg ephedrine

Emergence
- assessment of exit phase by
eye opening, head lifting,
hand grip influenced by
disease process
- use of short acting
non-depolarizing agent
should obviate need for
anticholinesterase

Post-op
- HDU
- automatic chest physiotherapy
- avoid sedatives (hypnotics or
opiates)
- anticipate and treat infections
vigorously
- monitor oxygen saturation

Appendix 3

The myotonic dystrophy care card
(courtesy of Dr. Douglas Wilcox, Glasgow)

Available from the Scottish
Muscle Network
(www.gla.ac.uk/muscle/dm.htm),
based on information from the
the Scottish and Welsh Centres
and the Myotonic Dystrophy
Support Group. Region specific
versions are available.

The A4 sheet can be printed
off the website and folded to
fit a plastic wallet (details also
available from the above web
address).

CARE CARD

MYOTONIC DYSTROPHY

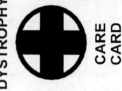

MEDICAL ALERT

The bearer of this card has **MYOTONIC DYSTROPHY**, a neuromuscular condition that may cause the following:

A. muscle weakness and stiffness.

B. extreme tiredness.

C. speech difficulties.

D. Adverse reaction to commonly used anaesthetic agents.

E. Abnormal heart rhythm.

Personal Details

Name

DoB

Address

Phone

Emergency Contact

Name

Address

Phone

Version 9.03/.dtf: 14/01/02

Page 3

Further Information

Cardiff Muscular Dystrophy Centre:
Consultant: Professor Harper, Dr Mark Rogers, Secretary: Leah Bartlett
Tel: 0292 074 4021

Myotonic Dystrophy Support Group:
a self help group, willing to provide support to families affected by Myotonic Dystrophy.
Tel: 0115 987 0080
Email: mdsg@tesco.net
Web: www.mdsguk.org

Muscular Dystrophy Campaign:
a charity funding medical research and support, including Family Care Officers, for people with neuromuscular conditions.
Tel: 0007 720 8055
Email: info@muscular-dystrophy.org
Web: www.muscular-dystrophy.org

Scottish Muscle Network:
information about local and updated versions of the Card are: www.gla.ac.uk/muscle/dm.htm
Card enquiries and suggestions to:
D.E.Wilcox@clinmed.gla.ac.uk

Page 2

Myotonic Dystrophy and how it could affect your health.

Tiredness:
Tiredness is very common and can occur at any time of the day. Sometimes it can be extreme.

Muscle weakness:
Weakness is very variable and can range from mild to severe. It is particularly involves the face and eyelids, jaw, neck, forearms and hands, lower legs and feet. It can affect speech and give lack of facial expression.

Myotonic:
Myotonia is a difficulty in relaxing a muscle after it has been contracted, e.g. after gripping something, it might be difficult to let go.

Heart problems:
Abnormal rhythm of the heart might require treatment. This can affect adults, even those without symptoms.
Regular ECGs (heart tracings) of affected adults are advised to detect problems at an early stage.

Chest and breathing problems:
Chest infections may result from weakness of breathing muscles, including the diaphragm, or from inadequate breathing during the night might lead to disturbed sleep, snoring, difficulty waking, morning headaches and daytime sleepiness.

Digestive problems:
These are common as the muscle throughout the digestive system may be affected. This may lead to: swallowing problems (which can also be a cause of food entering the lungs), pains in the bowels with constipation and diarrhea, soiling of underwear particularly when stressed or excited and occasionally enlargement of the large bowel.
Gallstones, which can cause painful spasms after eating fatty food, can be a problem in myotonic dystrophy even in young adults and great care needs to be taken with any surgical treatment.

Eye problems:
Cataracts can cause blurring and dimming of vision. This may be the only problem caused by myotonic dystrophy, particularly in the first affected generation of a family. Droopy eyelids can cause a problem with reading and watching television. You should have regular checks at the opticians and see a medical eye specialist if there is any concern.

Anaesthetics and surgery:
Myotonic dystrophy can cause problems with your recovery after an operation when certain anaesthetic drugs are used. Make sure the surgeon and anaesthetist know about your myotonic dystrophy before an operation. They may wish to contact a specialist centre for advice. Carry this document or an Alert Card in your wallet or purse at all times, in case of an accident or emergency.

Other problems include:
Diabetes, (ask to have your blood or urine sugar checked), male infertility, the muscle in the womb can be involved and lead to long difficult labour (possibly with bleeding afterwards), and obstetric help may be required. The brain can be affected causing thinking and learning difficulty, especially when onset is in childhood. Personality changes can include awkwardness and liking a "set routine".

Special difficulties in affected children:
Muscle involvement can be more severe, especially when myotonic dystrophy is present at birth. Sometimes severely affected babies may live only a short time. If an affected baby survives infancy, parents and doctors are often surprised by the good progress the child subsequently makes but speech, educational and behavioural problems can occur.

Inheritance:
Other family members are frequently affected. It can affect and be passed on by both sexes, but women are at risk of having a seriously affected child.
Genetic counselling is advised if genetic testing is being considered.
Accurate genetic tests are possible, for healthy people who are at risk of developing myotonic dystrophy because they have an affected relative and in early pregnancy where one parent is affected.

Page 1

Bibliography

Further reading for patients and families

Emery, E. A. H. (2000) *Muscular dystrophy. The facts* (2nd edn). Oxford University Press, Oxford.

This clearly written book, in the same series as the present volume, deals mainly with the severe Duchenne form of muscular dystrophy, but contains valuable details on muscle disease in general. It also gives a fuller listing of muscular dystrophy organizations, which could be helpful for patients in countries without a specific support group for myotonic dystrophy.

Harper, P. S. (2001) *Myotonic dystrophy* (3rd edn). Saunders, London.

A book written for professionals, but despite this, some patients have found it helpful. It is expensive, so perhaps best bought by your doctor or clinic!

Harper, P. S. (2001) *Practical genetic counselling.* Butterworth-Heineman, Oxford.

The first part of this book covers the general aspects of genetic counselling and related areas.

Harpin, P. (2000) Muscular dystrophy. *Adaptations manual*. Muscular Dystrophy Campaign, London.

This provides valuable details on a wide range of aids and adaptations, many of which will be extremely useful for myotonic dystrophy patients, especially those with more marked muscle weakness. It is also available as a CD.

Iwakita, H. (2000) *Myotonic dystrophy*. Tokyo.

This book, written in Japanese, contains sections on disability aids and rehabilitation and will be valuable for patients and their doctors living in Japan.

Jennekens, F., De Die-Smulders, C., Busch, H., and Höweler, C. J. (2001) *Myotone dystrofie*. Elsevier, Amsterdam.

This book is written in Dutch, specifically for patients and families, and should be very valuable for anyone living in the Netherlands or neighbouring regions.

More specialized references on various aspects; mainly useful for professionals

Early descriptions

Batten, F. E. and Gibb, H. P. (1909) Myotonia atrophica. *Brain* **32**, 187–205.

Steinert, H. (1909) Myopathologische Beiträge 1. über das klinische und anatomische Bild des Muskelschwunds der Myotoniker. *Dtsch. Z. Nervenheilkd.* **37**, 58–104.

Vanier, T. M. (1960) Dystrophia myotonica in childhood. *BMJ* **2**, 1284–8.

Course of the disorder

Mathieu, J., De Braekeleer, M., Prévost, C. *et al.* (1992) Myotonic dystrophy: clinical assessment of muscular disability in an isolated population with presumed homogeneous mutation. *Neurology* **42**, 203–8.

Related disorders

Day, J. W., Roelofs, R., Leroy, B. *et al.* (1999) Clinical and genetic characteristics of a five-generation family with a novel form of myotonic dystrophy (DM2). *Neuromusc. Disord.* **9**, 19–27.

Karpati, G., Griggs, R. C., and Hilton-Jones, D. (ed.) (2001) *Disorders of Voluntary Muscle* (7th edn). Cambridge University Press, Cambridge.

Ricker, K., Koch, M. C., Lehmann-Horn, F. *et al.* (1994) Proximal myotonic myopathy; a new dominant disorder with myotonia, muscle weakness and cataracts. *Neurology* **44**, 1448–52.

Smooth muscle

Brunner, H. G., Hamel, B. G. C., Rieu, P. *et al.* (1992) Intestinal pseudo-obstruction in myotonic dystrophy. *J. Med. Genet.* **29**, 791–3.

Goldberg, H. I. and Sheft, D. J. (1972) Esophageal and colon changes in myotonia dystrophica. *Gastroenterology* **63**, 134–9.

Ronnblom, A., Forsberg, H., and Danielsson, A. (1996) Gastrointestinal symptoms in myotonic dystrophy. *Scand. J. Gastroenterol.* **31**, 654–7.

Heart, lung, and anaesthetic problems

Aldridge, L. M. (1985) Anaesthetic problems in myotonic dystrophy—a case report and review of the Aberdeen experience comprising 48 general anaesthetics in a further 16 patients. *Br. J. Anaesth.* **57**, 1119–30.

Gilmartin, J. J., Cooper, B. G., Griffiths, C. J. *et al.* (1991) Breathing during sleep in patients with myotonic dystrophy and non-myotonic respiratory muscle weakness. Q. J. Med. **78**, 21–31.

Lazarus, A., Varin, J., Ounnoughene, Z. et al. (1999) Relationships among electrophysiological findings and clinical status, heart function, and extent of DNA mutation in myotonic dystrophy. Circulation **99**, 1041–6.

Mathieu, J., Allard, P., Gobeil, G. et al. (1997) Anaesthetic and surgical complications in 219 cases of myotonic dystrophy. Neurology **49**, 646–50.

Phillips, M. F. and Harper, P. S. (1997) Cardiac disease in myotonic dystrophy. Cardiovasc. Res. **33**, 13–22.

Somnolence and related problems

Censori, B., Provinciali, L., Danni, M. et al. (1994) Brain involvement in myotonic dystrophy: MRI features and their relationship to clinical and cognitive conditions. Acta Neurol. Scand. **90**, 211–17.

Phillips, M. F., Steer, H. M., Soldan, J. R. et al. (1999) Daytime somnolence in myotonic dystrophy. J. Neurol. **246**, 275–82.

Rubinsztein, J. S., Rubinsztein, D. C., Goodburn, S. et al. (1998) Apathy and hypersomnia are common features of myotonic dystrophy. J. Neurol. Neurosurg. Psychiat. **64**, 510–15.

Hormones

Morrone, A., Pegoraro, E., Angelini, C. et al. (1997) RNA metabolism in myotonic dystrophy: patient muscle shows decreased insulin receptor RNA and protein consistent with abnormal insulin resistance. J Clin Invest **99**, 1691–8.

Vazquez, J. A., Pinies, J. A., Martual, P. et al. (1990) Hypothalmic–pituitary testicular function in 70 patients with myotonic dystrophy. *J. Endocrinol. Invest.* **13**, 375–9.

Childhood myotonic dystrophy

De Die-Smulders, C. (2000) Long-term clinical and genetic studies in myotonic dystrophy. Thesis, University of Maastricht.

Hageman, A. T., Gabreels, F. J., Liem, K. D. *et al.* (1993) Congenital myotonic dystrophy: a report on thirteen cases and a review of the literature. *J. Neurol. Sci.* **115**, 95–101.

Genetic aspects

Brook, J. D., McCurrach, M. E., Harley, H. G. *et al.* (1992) Molecular basis of myotonic dystrophy: expansion of a trinucleotide (CTG) repeat at the 3′ end of a transcript encoding a protein kinase family member. *Cell* **68**, 799–808.

Fokstuen, S., Myring, J., Evans, C. *et al.* (2001) Presymptomatic testing in myotonic dystrophy: genetic counselling approaches. *J. Med. Genet.* **38**, 846–50.

Harper, P. S., Harley, H. G., Reardon, W. *et al.* (1992) Anticipation in myotonic dystrophy: new light on an old problem. *Am J Hum Genet* **51**, 10–16.

Höweler, C. J., Busch, H. F. M., Geraedts, J. P. M. *et al.* (1989) Anticipation in myotonic dystrophy: fact or fiction? *Brain* **112**, 779–97.

Liquori, C., Ricker, K., Moseley, M. L. *et al.* (2001) Myotonic Dystrophy type 2 caused by a CCTG expansion in intron 1 of ZNF9. *Science* **293**, 864–7.

Mankodi, A., Logigian, E., Callahan, L. *et al.* (2000) Myotonic dystrophy in transgenic mice expressing an expanded CUG repeat. *Science* **289**, 1769–73.

Bibliography

Mathieu, J., De Braekeleer, M., and Prévost, C. (1990) Geneaological reconstruction of myotonic dystrophy in the Saguenay-Lac-Saint-Jean area (Quebec, Canada). *Neurology* **40**, 839–42.

Management

Harper, P. S., Van Engelen, B. G. M., Eymard, B., and Wilcox, D. (2002) Myotonic dystrophy: present management, future therapy. *Neuromusc. Disord.* (in press).

Index

Index

Index